Malnutrition and Nutrient Deficiency

Malnutrition and Nutrient Deficiency

Edited by
Clara Nesbit

Larsen & Keller
www.larsen-keller.com

Malnutrition and Nutrient Deficiency
Edited by Clara Nesbit
ISBN: 978-1-63549-699-4 (Hardback)

Larsen & Keller
Published by Larsen and Keller Education,
5 Penn Plaza,
19th Floor,
New York, NY 10001, USA

Cataloging-in-Publication Data

Malnutrition and nutrient deficiency / edited by Clara Nesbit.
p. cm.
Includes bibliographical references and index.
ISBN 978-1-63549-699-4
1. Malnutrition. 2. Nutrition disorders. 3. Deficiency diseases.
I. Nesbit, Clara.
RA645.N87 M35 2018
363.8--dc23

Printed and bound in China.

For more information regarding Larsen and Keller Education and its products, please visit the publisher's website www.larsen-keller.com

Table of Contents

Preface

One of the world's most crucial problem today is malnutrition and nutrient deficiency, especially in children. Lack of basic food and water resources, coupled with poverty has led to an increase in this issue worldwide. Malnutrition refers to the state of having nutrition deficiency from not eating enough or enough nutrition rich food. It also includes lack of vitamins, carbohydrates, minerals, proteins and even calories. This book presents the subject of malnutrition and nutrient deficiency as easy and informative as possible, for the readers. The textbook also includes topics dealing with cause and effect of this problem. This book, with its detailed analyses and data, will prove immensely beneficial to professionals and students involved in this area at various levels.

A foreword of all chapters of the book is provided below:

Chapter 1 - Malnutrition is a condition caused by the lack of intake of nutrition, such as calories, vitamins, etc. Protein-energy malnutrition causes disorders like kwashiorkor, stunted growth and marasmus. This is an introductory chapter which will introduce briefly all the significant aspects of malnutrition; **Chapter 2 -** Overnutrition is caused by excessive intake of nutrients. Excess of nutrients can lead to iron poisoning. Being overweight and hypervitaminosis are some complications related to overnutrition. The topics elaborated in this chapter will help in gaining a better perspective about the concept of overnutrition; **Chapter 3 -** Nutritional deficiencies can be of many types like vitamin A deficiency, vitamin E deficiency, vitamin K deficiency and vitamin D deficiency as well as deficiencies which lead to malnutrition such as iodine deficiency, zinc deficiency, hypocalcaemia, mineral deficiency, etc. The aspects elucidated in this section are of vital importance, and provide a better understanding of nutritional deficiencies; **Chapter 4 -** Malnutrition is the deficiency or surplus of nutrients in the body. The effects of malnutrition are Wernicke-Korsakoff syndrome, stunted growth, wasting, rickets, anemia, pellagra and beriberi. The aspects elucidated in this chapter are of vital importance, and provide a better understanding of the effects of malnutrition.

At the end, I would like to thank all the people associated with this book devoting their precious time and providing their valuable contributions to this book. I would also like to express my gratitude to my fellow colleagues who encouraged me throughout the process.

Editor

1

Malnutrition and its Types

Malnutrition is a condition caused by the lack of intake of nutrition, such as calories, vitamins, etc. Protein-energy malnutrition causes disorders like kwashiorkor, stunted growth and marasmus. This is an introductory chapter which will introduce briefly all the significant aspects of malnutrition.

Malnutrition

Malnutrition is a condition that results from eating a diet in which nutrients are either not enough or are too much such that the diet causes health problems. It may involve calories, protein, carbohydrates, vitamins or minerals. Not enough nutrients is called undernutrition or undernourishment while too much is called overnutrition. Malnutrition is often used to specifically refer to undernutrition where an individual is not getting enough calories, protein, or micronutrients. If undernutrition occurs during pregnancy, or before two years of age, it may result in permanent problems with physical and mental development. Extreme undernourishment, known as starvation, may have symptoms that include: a short height, thin body, very poor energy levels, and swollen legs and abdomen. People also often get infections and are frequently cold. The symptoms of micronutrient deficiencies depend on the micronutrient that is lacking.

Undernourishment is most often due to not enough high-quality food being available to eat. This is often related to high food prices and poverty. A lack of breastfeeding may contribute, as may a number of infectious diseases such as: gastroenteritis, pneumonia, malaria, and measles, which increase nutrient requirements. There are two main types of undernutrition: protein-energy malnutrition and dietary deficiencies. Protein-energy malnutrition has two severe forms: marasmus (a lack of protein and calories) and kwashiorkor (a lack of just protein). Common micronutrient deficiencies include: a lack of iron, iodine, and vitamin A. During pregnancy, due to the body's increased need, deficiencies may become more common. In some developing countries, overnutrition in the form of obesity is beginning to present within the same communities as undernutrition. Other causes of malnutrition include anorexia nervosa and bariatric surgery.

Efforts to improve nutrition are some of the most effective forms of development aid. Breastfeeding can reduce rates of malnutrition and death in children, and efforts to promote the practice increase the rates of breastfeeding. In young children, providing food (in addition to breastmilk) between six months and two years of age improves outcomes.

There is also good evidence supporting the supplementation of a number of micronutrients to women during pregnancy and among young children in the developing world. To get food to people who need it most, both delivering food and providing money so people can buy food within local markets are effective. Simply feeding students at school is insufficient. Management of severe malnutrition within the person's home with ready-to-use therapeutic foods is possible much of the time. In those who have severe malnutrition complicated by other health problems, treatment in a hospital setting is recommended. This often involves managing low blood sugar and body temperature, addressing dehydration, and gradual feeding. Routine antibiotics are usually recommended due to the high risk of infection. Longer-term measures include: improving agricultural practices, reducing poverty, improving sanitation, and the empowerment of women.

There were 793 million undernourished people in the world in 2015 (13% of the total population). This is a reduction of 216 million people since 1990 when 23% were undernourished. In 2012 it was estimated that another billion people had a lack of vitamins and minerals. In 2015, protein-energy malnutrition was estimated to have resulted in 323,000 deaths—down from 510,000 deaths in 1990. Other nutritional deficiencies, which include iodine deficiency and iron deficiency anemia, result in another 83,000 deaths. In 2010, malnutrition was the cause of 1.4% of all disability adjusted life years. About a third of deaths in children are believed to be due to undernutrition, although the deaths are rarely labelled as such. In 2010, it was estimated to have contributed to about 1.5 million deaths in women and children, though some estimate the number may be greater than 3 million. An additional 165 million children were estimated to have stunted growth from malnutrition in 2013. Undernutrition is more common in developing countries. Certain groups have higher rates of undernutrition, including women—in particular while pregnant or breastfeeding—children under five years of age, and the elderly. In the elderly, undernutrition becomes more common due to physical, psychological, and social factors.

Definitions

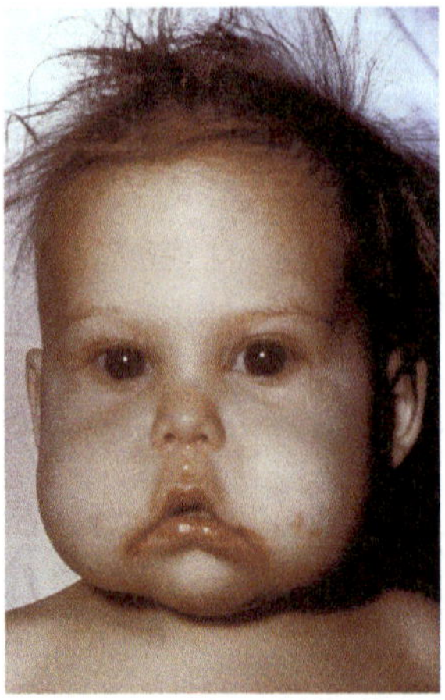

Child in the United States with signs of Kwashiorkor, a dietary protein deficiency.

Unless specifically mentioned otherwise, the term malnutrition refers to undernutrition for the remainder of this lesson. Malnutrition can be divided into two different types, SAM and MAM. SAM refers to children with severe acute malnutrition. MAM refers to moderate acute malnutrition.

Undernutrition and Overnutrition

Malnutrition is caused by eating a diet in which nutrients are *not enough* or are *too much* such that it causes health problems. It is a category of diseases that includes undernutrition and overnutrition. Overnutrition can result in obesity and being overweight. In some developing countries, overnutrition in the form of obesity is beginning to present within the same communities as undernutrition.

However, the term malnutrition is commonly used to refer to undernutrition only. This applies particularly to the context of development cooperation. Therefore, "malnutrition" in documents by the World Health Organization, UNICEF, Save the Children or other international non-governmental organizations (NGOs) usually is equated to undernutrition.

Protein-energy Malnutrition

Undernutrition is sometimes used as a synonym of protein–energy malnutrition (PEM). While other include both micronutrient deficiencies and protein energy malnutrition in its definition. It differs from calorie restriction in that calorie restriction may not result in negative health effects. The term hypoalimentation means underfeeding.

The term "severe malnutrition" or "severe undernutrition" is often used to refer specifically to PEM. PEM is often associated with micronutrient deficiency. Two forms of PEM are kwashiorkor and marasmus, and they commonly coexist.

Kwashiorkor

Kwashiorkor ('displaced child') is mainly caused by inadequate protein intake resulting in a low concentration of amino acids. The main symptoms are edema, wasting, liver enlargement, hypoalbuminaemia, steatosis, and possibly depigmentation of skin and hair. Kwashiorkor is identified by swelling of the extremities and belly, which is deceiving of actual nutritional status.

Marasmus

Marasmus ('to waste away') is caused by an inadequate intake of protein and energy. The main symptoms are severe wasting, leaving little or no edema, minimal subcutaneous fat, severe muscle wasting, and non-normal serum albumin levels. Marasmus can result from a sustained diet of inadequate energy and protein, and the metabolism adapts to prolong survival. It is traditionally seen in famine, significant food restriction, or more severe cases of anorexia. Conditions are characterized by extreme wasting of the muscles and a gaunt expression.

Undernutrition, Hunger

Undernutrition encompasses stunted growth (stunting), wasting, and deficiencies of essential vitamins and minerals (collectively referred to as micronutrients). The term hunger, which describes a feeling of discomfort from not eating, has been used to describe undernutrition, especially in reference to food insecurity.

Definition by Gomez

In 1956, Gómez and Galvan studied factors associated with death in a group of malnourished (undernourished) children in a hospital in Mexico City, Mexico and defined categories of malnutrition: first, second, and third degree. The degrees were based on weight below a specified percentage of median weight for age. The risk of death increases with increasing degree of malnutrition. An adaptation of Gomez's original classification is still used today. While it provides a way to compare malnutrition within and between populations, the classification has been criticized for being "arbitrary" and for not considering overweight as a form of malnutrition. Also, height alone may not be the best indicator of malnutrition; children who are born prematurely may be considered short for their age even if they have good nutrition.

Degree of PEM	% of desired body weight for age and sex
Normal	90%-100%
Mild: Grade I (1st degree)	75%-89%
Moderate: Grade II (2nd degree)	60%-74%
Severe: Grade III (3rd degree)	<60%

Definition by Waterlow

John Conrad Waterlow established a new classification for malnutrition. Instead of using just weight for age measurements, the classification established by Waterlow combines weight-for-height (indicating acute episodes of malnutrition) with height-for-age to show the stunting that results from chronic malnutrition. One advantage of the Waterlow classification over the Gomez classification is that weight for height can be examined even if ages are not known.

Degree of PEM	Stunting (%) Height for age	Wasting (%) Weight for height
Normal: Grade 0	>95%	>90%
Mild: Grade I	87.5-95%	80-90%
Moderate: Grade II	80-87.5%	70-80%
Severe: Grade III	<80%	<70%

These classifications of malnutrition are commonly used with some modifications by WHO.

Effects

Malnutrition increases the risk of infection and infectious disease, and moderate malnutrition weakens every part of the immune system. For example, it is a major risk factor in the onset of active tuberculosis. Protein and energy malnutrition and deficiencies of specific micronutrients (including iron, zinc, and vitamins) increase susceptibility to infection. Malnutrition affects HIV transmission by increasing the risk of transmission from mother to child and also increasing replication of the virus. In communities or areas that lack access to safe drinking water, these additional health risks present a critical problem. Lower energy and impaired function of the brain also represent the downward spiral of malnutrition as victims are less able to perform the tasks they need to in order to acquire food, earn an income, or gain an education.

Vitamin-deficiency-related diseases (such as scurvy and rickets).

Hypoglycemia (low blood sugar) can result from a child not eating for 4 to 6 hours. Hypoglycemia should be considered if there is lethargy, limpness, convulsion, or loss of consciousness. If blood sugar can be measured immediately and quickly, perform a finger or heel stick.

Signs

In those with malnutrition some of the signs of dehydration differ. Children; however, may still be interested in drinking, have decreased interactions with the world around them, have decreased urine output, and may be cool to touch.

Site	Sign
Face	Moon face (kwashiorkor), simian facies (marasmus)
Eye	Dry eyes, pale conjunctiva, Bitot's spots (vitamin A), periorbital edema
Mouth	Angular stomatitis, cheilitis, glossitis, spongy bleeding gums (vitamin C), parotid enlargement
Teeth	Enamel mottling, delayed eruption
Hair	Dull, sparse, brittle hair, hypopigmentation, flag sign (alternating bands of light and normal color), broomstick eyelashes, alopecia
Skin	Loose and wrinkled (marasmus), shiny and edematous (kwashiorkor), dry, follicular hyperkeratosis, patchy hyper- and hypopigmentation, erosions, poor wound healing
Nail	Koilonychia, thin and soft nail plates, fissures or ridges
Musculature	Muscles wasting, particularly in the buttocks and thighs
Skeletal	Deformities usually a result of calcium, vitamin D, or vitamin C deficiencies

Abdomen	Distended - hepatomegaly with fatty liver, ascites may be present
Cardiovascular	Bradycardia, hypotension, reduced cardiac output, small vessel vasculopathy
Neurologic	Global development delay, loss of knee and ankle reflexes, poor memory
Hematological	Pallor, petechiae, bleeding diathesis
Behavior	Lethargic, apathetic

Cognitive Development

Protein-calorie malnutrition can cause cognitive impairments. For humans, "critical period varies from the final third of gestation to the first 2 years of life". Iron deficiency anemia in children under two years of age likely affects brain function acutely and probably also chronically. Folate deficiency has been linked to neural tube defects.

Malnutrition in the form of iodine deficiency is "the most common preventable cause of mental impairment worldwide." "Even moderate deficiency, especially in pregnant women and infants, lowers intelligence by 10 to 15 I.Q. points, shaving incalculable potential off a nation's development. The most visible and severe effects — disabling goiters, cretinism and dwarfism — affect a tiny minority, usually in mountain villages. But 16 percent of the world's people have at least mild goiter, a swollen thyroid gland in the neck."

Causes

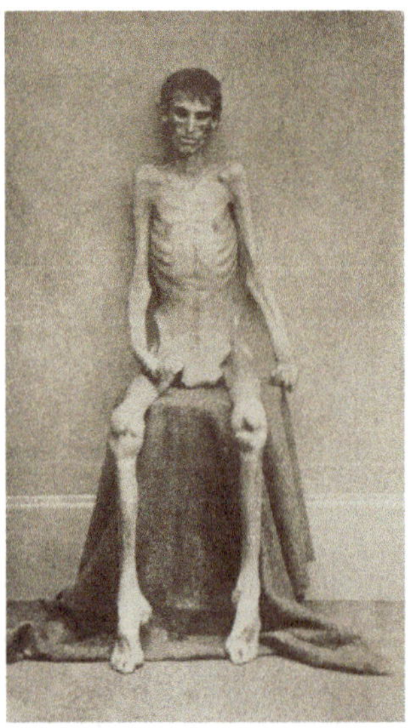

Union Army soldier on his release from Andersonville prison, 1865

Major causes of malnutrition include poverty and food prices, dietary practices and agricultural productivity, with many individual cases being a mixture of several factors. Clinical malnutrition, such as in cachexia, is a major burden also in developed countries. Various scales of analysis also have to be considered in order to determine the sociopolitical causes of malnutrition. For example, the population of a community may be at risk if the area lacks health-related services, but on a smaller scale certain households or individuals may be at even higher risk due to differences in income levels, access to land, or levels of education.

Diseases

Malnutrition can be a consequence of health issues such as gastroenteritis or chronic illness, especially the HIV/AIDS pandemic. Diarrhea and other infections can cause malnutrition through decreased nutrient absorption, decreased intake of food, increased metabolic requirements, and direct nutrient loss. Parasite infections, in particular intestinal worm infections (helminthiasis), can also lead to malnutrition. A leading cause of diarrhea and intestinal worm infections in children in developing countries is lack of sanitation and hygiene.

People may become malnourished due to abnormal nutrient loss (due to diarrhea or chronic illness affecting the small bowel). This conditions may include Crohn's disease or untreated coeliac disease. Malnutrition may also occur due to increased energy expenditure (secondary malnutrition).

Dietary Practices

Undernutrition

A lack of adequate breastfeeding leads to malnutrition in infants and children, associated with the deaths of an estimated one million children annually. Illegal advertising of breast milk substitutes continues three decades after its 1981 prohibition under the *WHO International Code of Marketing Breast Milk Substitutes.*

Deriving too much of one's diet from a single source, such as eating almost exclusively corn or rice, can cause malnutrition. This may either be from a lack of education about proper nutrition, or from only having access to a single food source.

It is not just the total amount of calories that matters but specific nutritional deficiencies such as vitamin A deficiency, iron deficiency or zinc deficiency can also increase risk of death.

Overnutrition

Overnutrition caused by overeating is also a form of malnutrition. In the United States, more than half of all adults are now overweight — a condition that, like hunger, increases susceptibility to disease and disability, reduces worker productivity, and lowers life expectancy. Overeating is much more common in the United States, where for the majority of people, access to food is not an issue. Many parts of the world have access to a surplus of non-nutritious food, in addition to increased sedentary lifestyles. Yale psychologist Kelly Brownell calls this a "toxic food environment" where fat and sugar laden foods have taken precedence over healthy nutritious foods.

The issue in these developed countries is choosing the right kind of food. More fast food is consumed per capita in the United States than in any other country. The reason for this mass consumption of fast food is its affordability and accessibility. Often fast food, low in cost and nutrition, is high in calories and heavily promoted. When these eating habits are combined with increasingly urbanized, automated, and more sedentary lifestyles, it becomes clear why weight gain is difficult to avoid.

Not only does obesity occur in developed countries, problems are also occurring in developing countries in areas where income is on the rise. Overeating is also a problem in countries where hunger and poverty persist. In China, consumption of high-fat foods has increased while consumption of rice and other goods has decreased.

Overeating leads to many diseases, such as heart disease and diabetes, that may result in death.

Poverty and Food Prices

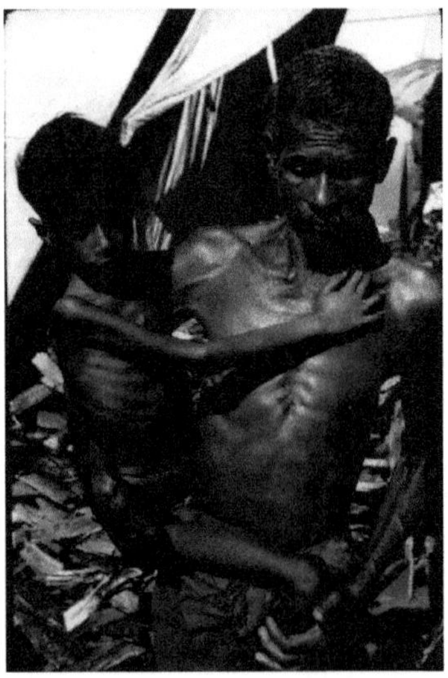

A child with extreme malnutrition

In Bangladesh, poor socioeconomic position was associated with chronic malnutrition since it inhibits purchase of nutritious foods such as milk, meat, poultry, and fruits. As much as food shortages may be a contributing factor to malnutrition in countries with lack of technology, the FAO (Food and Agriculture Organization) has estimated that eighty percent of malnourished children living in the developing world live in countries that produce food surpluses. The economist Amartya Sen observed that, in recent decades, famine has always been a problem of food distribution and/or poverty, as there has been sufficient food to feed the whole population of the world. He states that malnutrition and famine were more related to problems of food distribution and purchasing power.

It is argued that commodity speculators are increasing the cost of food. As the real estate bubble in the United States was collapsing, it is said that trillions of dollars moved to invest in food and primary commodities, causing the 2007–2008 food price crisis.

The use of biofuels as a replacement for traditional fuels and raises the price of food. The United Nations special rapporteur on the right to food, Jean Ziegler proposes that agricultural waste, such as corn cobs and banana leaves, rather than crops themselves be used as fuel.

Agricultural Productivity

Local food shortages can be caused by a lack of arable land, adverse weather, lower farming skills such as crop rotation, or by a lack of technology or resources needed for the higher yields found in modern agriculture, such as fertilizers, pesticides, irrigation, machinery and storage facilities. As a result of widespread poverty, farmers cannot afford or governments cannot provide the resources necessary to improve local yields. The World Bank and some wealthy donor countries also press nations that depend on aid to cut or eliminate subsidized agricultural inputs such as fertilizer, in the name of free market policies even as the United States and Europe extensively subsidized their own farmers. Many, if not most, farmers cannot afford fertilizer at market prices, leading to low agricultural production and wages and high, unaffordable food prices. Reasons for the unavailability of fertilizer include moves to stop supplying fertilizer on environmental grounds, cited as the obstacle to feeding Africa by the Green Revolution pioneers Norman Borlaug and Keith Rosenberg.

Future Threats

There are a number of potential disruptions to global food supply that could cause widespread malnutrition.

Climate change is of importance to food security, with 95 percent of all malnourished peoples living in the relatively stable climate region of the sub-tropics and tropics. According to the latest IPCC reports, temperature increases in these regions are "very likely." Even small changes in temperatures can lead to increased frequency of extreme weather conditions. Many of these have great impact on agricultural production and hence nutrition. For example, the 1998–2001 central Asian drought brought about an 80 percent livestock loss and 50 percent reduction in wheat and barley crops in Iran. Similar figures were present in other nations. An increase in extreme weather such as drought in regions such as Sub-Saharan Africa would have even greater consequences in terms of malnutrition. Even without an increase of extreme weather events, a simple increase in temperature reduces the productivity of many crop species, also decreasing food security in these regions.

Colony collapse disorder is a phenomenon where bees die in large numbers. Since many agricultural crops worldwide are pollinated by bees, this represents a threat to the supply of food.

An epidemic of wheat stem rust caused by race Ug99 is currently spreading across Africa and into Asia and, it is feared, could wipe out more than 80 percent of the world's wheat crops.

Prevention

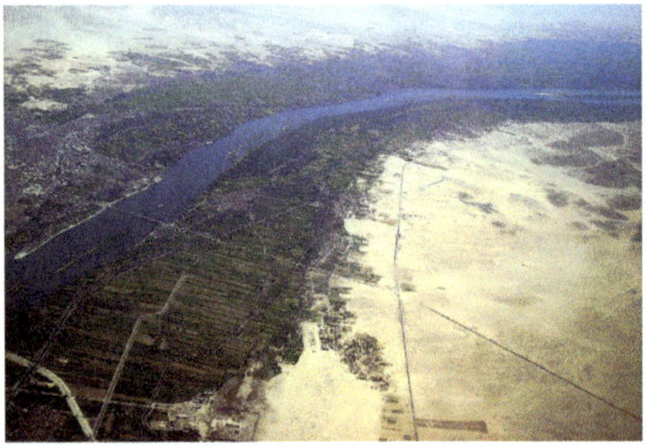

Irrigation canals have opened dry desert areas of Egypt to agriculture.

Food Security

The effort to bring modern agricultural techniques found in the West, such as nitrogen fertilizers and pesticides, to Asia, called the Green Revolution, resulted in decreases in malnutrition similar to those seen earlier in Western nations. This was possible because of existing infrastructure and institutions that are in short supply in Africa, such as a system of roads or public seed companies that made seeds available. Investments in agriculture, such as subsidized fertilizers and seeds, increases food harvest and reduces food prices. For example, in the case of Malawi, almost five million of its 13 million people used to need emergency food aid. However, after the government changed policy and subsidies for fertilizer and seed were introduced against World Bank strictures, farmers produced record-breaking corn harvests as production leaped to 3.4 million in 2007 from 1.2 million in 2005, making Malawi a major food exporter. This lowered food prices and increased wages for farm workers. Such investments in agriculture are still needed in other African countries like the Democratic Republic of the Congo. The country has one of the highest prevalence of malnutrition even though it is blessed with great agricultural potential John Ulimwengu explains in his article for D+C. Proponents for investing in agriculture include Jeffrey Sachs, who has championed the idea that wealthy countries should invest in fertilizer and seed for Africa's farmers.

New technology in agricultural production also has great potential to combat undernutrition. By improving agricultural yields, farmers could reduce poverty by increasing income as well as open up area for diversification of crops for household use. The World Bank itself claims to be part of the solution to malnutrition, asserting that the best way for countries to succeed in breaking the cycle of poverty and malnutrition is to build export-led economies that will give them the financial means to buy foodstuffs on the world market.

Breastfeeding

As of 2016 is estimated that about 821,000 deaths of children less than five years old could be prevented globally per year through more widespread breastfeeding.

Fortified Foods

Manufacturers are trying to fortify everyday foods with micronutrients that can be sold to consumers such as wheat flour for Beladi bread in Egypt or fish sauce in Vietnam and the iodization of salt.

For example, flour has been fortified with iron, zinc, folic acid and other B vitamins such as thiamine, riboflavin,niacin and vitamin B12.

World Population

Restricting population size is a proposed solution. Thomas Malthus argued that population growth could be controlled by natural disasters and voluntary limits through "moral restraint." Robert Chapman suggests that an intervention through government policies is a necessary ingredient of curtailing global population growth. However, there are many who believe that the world has more than enough resources to sustain its population. Instead, these theorists point to unequal distribution of resources and under- or unutilized arable land as the cause for malnutrition problems. For example, Amartya Sen advocates that, "no matter how a famine is caused, methods of breaking it call for a large supply of food in the public distribution system. This applies not only to organizing rationing and control, but also to undertaking work programmes and other methods of increasing purchasing power for those hit by shifts in exchange entitlements in a general inflationary situation."

Food Sovereignty

One suggested policy framework to resolve access issues is termed food sovereignty—the right of peoples to define their own food, agriculture, livestock, and fisheries systems, in contrast to having food largely subjected to international market forces. Food First is one of the primary think tanks working to build support for food sovereignty. Neoliberals advocate for an increasing role of the free market.

Health Facilities

Another possible long term solution would be to increase access to health facilities to rural parts of the world. These facilities could monitor undernourished children, act as supplemental food distribution centers, and provide education on dietary needs. These types of facilities have already proven very successful in countries such as Peru and Ghana.

Global Initiatives

In April 2012, the Food Assistance Convention was signed, the world's first legally binding international agreement on food aid. The May 2012 Copenhagen Consensus recommended that efforts to combat hunger and malnutrition should be the first priority for politicians and private sector philanthropists looking to maximize the effectiveness of aid spending. They put this ahead of other priorities, like the fight against malaria and AIDS.

The main global policy to reduce hunger and poverty are the Sustainable Development Goals. In particular Goal 2: Zero hunger sets globally agreed targets to end hunger, achieve food security and improved nutrition and promote sustainable agriculture. The partnership Compact2025, led by IFPRI with the involvement of UN organisations, NGOs and private foundations develops and disseminates evidence-based advice to politicians and other decision-makers aimed at ending hunger and undernutrition in the coming 10 years, by 2025.

The EndingHunger campaign is an online communication campaign aimed at raising awareness of the hunger problem. It has many worked through viral videos depicting celebrities voicing their anger about the large number of hungry people in the world. Another initiative focused on improving the hunger situation by improving nutrition is the Scaling up Nutrition movement (SUN). Started in 2010 this movement of people from governments, civil society, the United Nations, donors, businesses and researchers, publishes a yearly progress report on the changes in their 55 partner countries.

Management

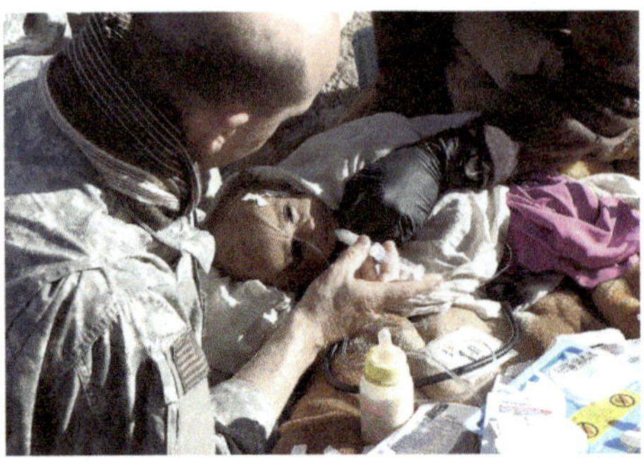

A malnourished Afghan child being treated by a medical team.

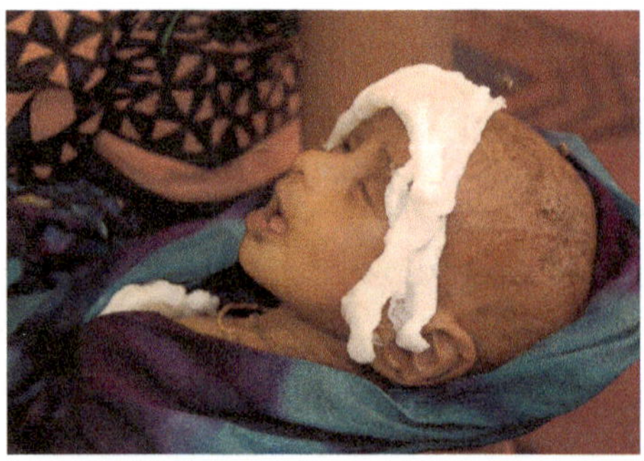

A Somali boy receiving treatment for malnourishment at a health facility.

In response to child malnutrition, the Bangladeshi government recommends ten steps for treating severe malnutrition. They are to prevent or treat dehydration, low blood sugar, low body temperature, infection, correct electrolyte imbalances and micronutrient deficiencies, start feeding cautiously, achieve catch-up growth, provide psychological support, and prepare for discharge and follow-up after recovery.

Among those patients who are hospitalized, nutritional support improves protein, colorie intake and weight.

Food

The evidence for benefit of supplementary feeding is poor. This is due to the small amount of research done on this treatment.

Specially formulated foods do however appear useful in those from the developing world with moderate acute malnutrition. In young children with severe acute malnutrition it is unclear if ready-to-use therapeutic food differs from a normal diet. They may have some benefits in humanitarian emergencies as they can be eaten directly from the packet, do not require refrigeration or mixing with clean water, and can be stored for years.

In those who are severely malnourished, feeding too much too quickly can result in refeeding syndrome. This can result regardless of route of feeding and can present itself a couple of days after eating with heart failure, dysrhythmias and confusion that can result in death.

Micronutrients

Treating malnutrition, mostly through fortifying foods with micronutrients (vitamins and minerals), improves lives at a lower cost and shorter time than other forms of aid, according to the World Bank. The Copenhagen Consensus, which look at a variety of development proposals, ranked micronutrient supplements as number one.

In those with diarrhea, once an initial four-hour rehydration period is completed, zinc supplementation is recommended. Daily zinc increases the chances of reducing the severity and duration of the diarrhea, and continuing with daily zinc for ten to fourteen days makes diarrhea less likely recur in the next two to three months.

In addition, malnourished children need both potassium and magnesium. This can be obtained by following the above recommendations for the dehydrated child to continue eating within two to three hours of starting rehydration, and including foods rich in potassium as above. Low blood potassium is worsened when base (as in Ringer's/Hartmann's) is given to treat acidosis without simultaneously providing potassium. As above, available home products such as salted and unsalted cereal water, salted and unsalted vegetable broth can be given early during the course of a child's diarrhea along with continued eating. Vitamin A, potassium, magnesium, and zinc should be added with other vitamins and minerals if available.

For a malnourished child with diarrhea from any cause, this should include foods rich in potassium such as bananas, green coconut water, and unsweetened fresh fruit juice.

Diarrhea

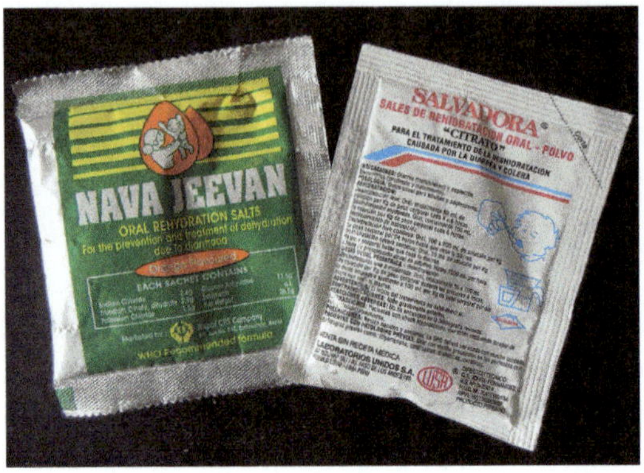

Examples of commercially available oral rehydration salts (Nepal on left, Peru on right).

The World Health Organization (WHO) recommends rehydrating a severely undernourished child who has diarrhea relatively slowly. The preferred method is with fluids by mouth using a drink called oral rehydration solution (ORS). The oral rehydration solution is both slightly sweet and slightly salty and the one recommended in those with severe undernutrition should have half the usual sodium and greater potassium. Fluids by nasogastric tube may be use in those who do not drink. Intravenous fluids are recommended only in those who have significant dehydration due to their potential complications. These complications include congestive heart failure. Over time, ORS developed into ORT, or oral rehydration therapy, which focused on increasing fluids by supplying salts, carbohydrates, and water. This switch from type of fluid to amount of fluid was crucial in order to prevent dehydration from diarrhea.

Breast feeding and eating should resume as soon as possible. Drinks such as soft drinks, fruit juices, or sweetened teas are not recommended as they contain too much sugar and may worsen diarrhea. Broad spectrum antibiotics are recommended in all severely undernourished children with diarrhea requiring admission to hospital.

To prevent dehydration readily available fluids, preferably with a modest amount of sugars and salt such as vegetable broth or salted rice water, may be used. The drinking of additional clean water is also recommended. Once dehydration develops oral rehydration solutions are preferred. As much of these drinks as the person wants can be given, unless there are signs of swelling. If vomiting occurs, fluids can be paused for 5–10 minutes and then restarting more slowly. Vomiting rarely prevents rehydration as fluid are still absorbed and the vomiting rarely last long. A severely malnourished child with what appears to be dehydration but who has not had diarrhea should be treated as if they have an infection.

For babies a dropper or syringe without the needle can be used to put small amounts of fluid into the mouth; for children under 2, a teaspoon every one to two minutes; and for older children and adults, frequent sips directly from a cup. After the first two hours, rehydration should be continued at the same or slower rate, determined by how much fluid the child wants and any ongoing diarrheal loses. After the first two hours of rehydration it is recommended that to alternate between rehydration and food.

In 2003, WHO and UNICEF recommended a reduced-osmolarity ORS which still treats dehydration but also reduced stool volume and vomiting. Reduced-osmolarity ORS is the current standard ORS with reasonably wide availability. For general use, one packet of ORS (glucose sugar, salt, potassium chloride, and trisodium citrate) is added to one liter of water; however, for malnourished children it is recommended that one packet of ORS be added to two liters of water along with an extra 50 grams of sucrose sugar and some stock potassium solution.

Malnourished children have an excess of body sodium. Recommendations for home remedies agree with one liter of water (34 oz.) and 6 teaspoons sugar and disagree regarding whether it is then one teaspoon of salt added or only 1/2, with perhaps most sources recommending 1/2 teaspoon of added salt to one liter water.

Low Blood Sugar

Hypoglycemia, whether known or suspected, can be treated with a mixture of sugar and water. If the child is conscious, the initial dose of sugar and water can be given by mouth. If the child is unconscious, give glucose by intravenous or nasogastric tube. If seizures occur after despite glucose, rectal diazepam is recommended. Blood sugar levels should be re-checked on two hour intervals.

Hypothermia

Hypothermia can occur. To prevent or treat this, the child can be kept warm with covering including of the head or by direct skin-to-skin contact with the mother or father and then covering both parent and child. Prolonged bathing or prolonged medical exams should be avoided. Warming methods are usually most important at night.

Economics

There is a growing realization among aid groups that giving cash or cash vouchers instead of food is a cheaper, faster, and more efficient way to deliver help to the hungry, particularly in areas where food is available but unaffordable. The UN's World Food Program, the biggest non-governmental distributor of food, announced that it will begin distributing cash and vouchers instead of food in some areas, which Josette Sheeran, the WFP's executive director, described as a "revolution" in food aid. The aid agency Concern Worldwide is piloting a method through a mobile phone operator, Safaricom, which runs a money transfer program that allows cash to be sent from one part of the country to another.

However, for people in a drought living a long way from and with limited access to markets, delivering food may be the most appropriate way to help. Fred Cuny stated that "the chances of saving lives at the outset of a relief operation are greatly reduced when food is imported. By the time it arrives in the country and gets to people, many will have died." U.S. law, which requires buying food at home rather than where the hungry live, is inefficient because approximately half of what is spent goes for transport. Cuny further pointed out "studies of every recent famine have shown that food was available in-country — though not always in the immediate food deficit area" and "even though by local standards the prices are too high for the poor to purchase it, it would usually be cheaper for a donor to buy the hoarded food at the inflated price than to import it from abroad."

Ethiopia has been pioneering a program that has now become part of the World Bank's prescribed method for coping with a food crisis and had been seen by aid organizations as a model of how to best help hungry nations. Through the country's main food assistance program, the Productive Safety Net Program, Ethiopia has been giving rural residents who are chronically short of food, a chance to work for food or cash. Foreign aid organizations like the World Food Program were then able to buy food locally from surplus areas to distribute in areas with a shortage of food. Ethiopia been pioneering a program, and Brazil has established a recycling program for organic waste that benefits farmers, urban poor, and the city in general. City residents separate organic waste from their garbage, bag it, and then exchange it for fresh fruit and vegetables from local farmers. As a result, the country's waste is reduced and the urban poor get a steady supply of nutritious food.

Epidemiology

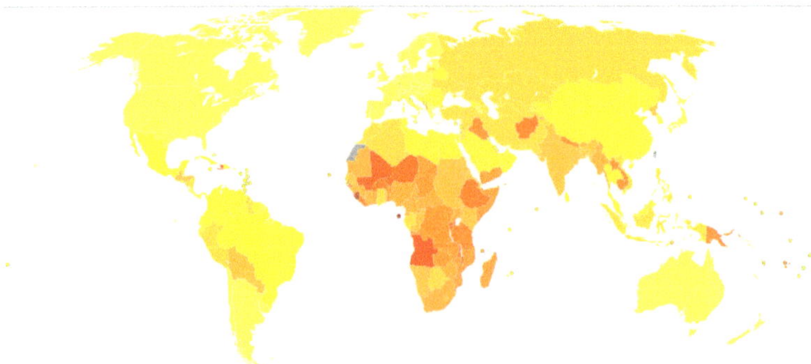

Disability-adjusted life year for nutritional deficiencies per 100,000 inhabitants in 2004. Nutritional deficiencies included: protein-energy malnutrition, iodine deficiency, vitamin A deficiency, and iron deficiency anaemia.

no data	400-600	1000-1200	1600-1800
<200	600-800	1200-1400	1800-2000
200-400	800-1000	1400-1600	2000-2200
			>2200

The figures provided on epidemiology all refer to *undernutrition* even if the term malnutrition is used which, by definition, could also apply to too much nutrition.

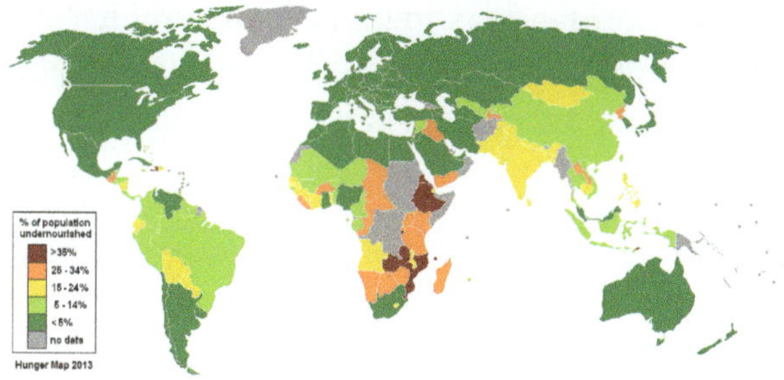

Percentage of population affected by undernutrition by country

People Affected

There were 793 million undernourished people in the world in 2015. This was 216 million fewer people than in 1990 when it was 991 million undernourished people. This is despite the world's farmers producing enough food to feed around 12 billion people – almost double the current world population.

Malnutrition, as of 2010, was the cause of 1.4% of all disability adjusted life years.

Number of undernourished globally							
Year	1970	1980	1990	1995	2005	2007/08	2014/16
Number in millions			843	788	848	923	793
Percentage in the developing world	37%	28%	20%		16%	17%	13.5%

Mortality

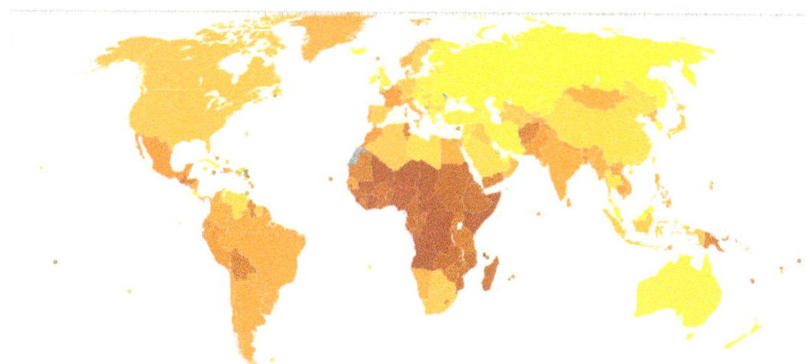

Deaths from nutritional deficiencies per million persons in 2012

0-4
5-8
9-13
14-23
24-34
35-56
57-91
92-220
221-365
366-1,207

Mortality due to malnutrition accounted for 58 percent of the total mortality in 2006: "In the world, approximately 62 million people, all causes of death combined, die each year. One in twelve people worldwide is malnourished and according to the Save the Children 2012 report, one in four of the world's children are chronically malnourished. In 2006, more than 36 million died of hunger or diseases due to deficiencies in micro-nutrients".

In 2010 protein-energy malnutrition resulted in 600,000 deaths down from 883,000 deaths in 1990. Other nutritional deficiencies, which include iodine deficiency and iron deficiency anemia, result in another 84,000 deaths. In 2010 malnutrition caused about 1.5 million deaths in women and children.

According to the World Health Organization, malnutrition is the biggest contributor to child mortality, present in half of all cases. Six million children die of hunger every year. Underweight births and intrauterine growth restrictions cause 2.2 million child deaths a year. Poor or non-existent breastfeeding causes another 1.4 million. Other deficiencies, such as lack of vitamin A or zinc, for example, account for 1 million. Malnutrition in the first two years is irreversible. Malnourished children grow up with worse health and lower education achievement. Their own children tend to be smaller. Malnutrition was previously seen as something that exacerbates the problems of diseases as measles, pneumonia and diarrhea. But malnutrition actually causes diseases and can be fatal in its own right.

Society and Culture

Roughly $300 million of aid goes to basic nutrition each year, less than $2 for each child below two in the 20 worst affected countries. In contrast, HIV/AIDS, which causes fewer deaths than child malnutrition, received $2.2 billion—$67 per person with HIV in all countries.

The International Crops Research Institute for the Semi-Arid Tropics (ICRISAT), a member of the CGIAR consortium, partners with farmers, governments, researchers and NGOs to help farmers grow nutritious crops, such as chickpea, groundnut, pigeonpea, millet and sorghum. This helps their communities have more balanced diets and become more resilient to pests and drought. The Harnessing Opportunities for Productivity Enhancement of Sorghum and Millets in Sub-Saharan Africa and the Indian-Subcontinent (HOPE) project, for example, is increasing yields of finger millet in Tanzania by encouraging farmers to grow improved varieties. Finger millet is very high in calcium, rich in iron and fiber, and has a better energy content than other cereals. These characteristics make it ideal for feeding to infants and the elderly.

Some organizations have begun working with teachers, policymakers, and managed food service contractors to mandate improved nutritional content and increased nutritional resources in school cafeterias from primary to university-level institutions. Health and nutrition have been proven to have close links with overall educational success.

The verb form is "malnourish"; "malnourishment" is sometimes used instead of "malnutrition."

Special Populations

Undernutrition is an important determinant of maternal and child health, accounting for more than a third of child deaths and more than 10 percent of the total global disease burden according to 2008 studies.

Children

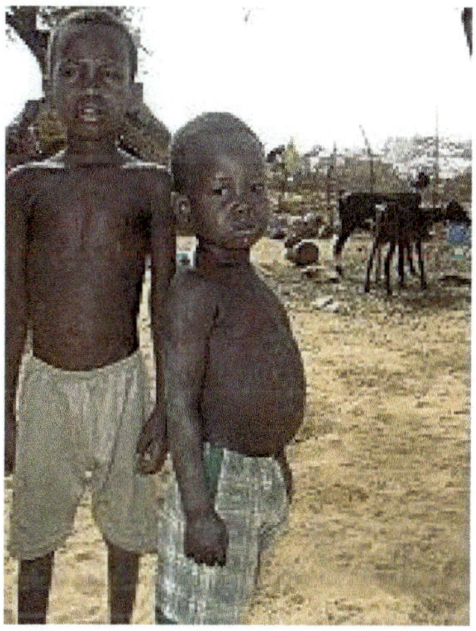

Malnourished children in Niger, during the 2005 famine.

The World Health Organization estimates that malnutrition accounts for 54 percent of child mortality worldwide, about 1 million children. Another estimate also by WHO states that childhood underweight is the cause for about 35% of all deaths of children under the age of five years worldwide.

As underweight children are more vulnerable to almost all infectious diseases, the *indirect* disease burden of malnutrition is estimated to be an order of magnitude higher than the disease burden of the *direct* effects of malnutrition. The combination of direct and indirect deaths from malnutrition caused by unsafe water, sanitation and hygiene (WASH) practices is estimated to lead to 860,000 deaths per year in children under five years of age.

Women

Gender

Researchers from the Centre for World Food Studies in 2003 found that the gap between levels of undernutrition in men and women is generally small, but that the gap varies from region to region and from country to country. These small-scale studies showed that female undernutrition prevalence rates exceeded male undernutrition prevalence rates in South/Southeast Asia and Latin America and were lower in Sub-Saharan Africa. Datasets for Ethiopia and Zimbabwe reported undernutrition rates between 1.5 and 2 times higher in men than in women; however, in India and

Pakistan, datasets rates of undernutrition were 1.5-2 times higher in women than in men. Intra-country variation also occurs, with frequent high gaps between regional undernutrition rates. Gender inequality in nutrition in some countries such as India is present in all stages of life.

Studies on nutrition concerning gender bias within households look at patterns of food allocation, and one study from 2003 suggested that women often receive a lower share of food requirements than men. Gender discrimination, gender roles, and social norms affecting women can lead to early marriage and childbearing, close birth spacing, and undernutrition, all of which contribute to malnourished mothers.

Within the household, there may be differences in levels of malnutrition between men and women, and these differences have been shown to vary significantly from one region to another, with problem areas showing relative deprivation of women. Samples of 1000 women in India in 2008 demonstrated that malnutrition in women is associated with poverty, lack of development and awareness, and illiteracy. The same study showed that gender discrimination in households can prevent a woman's access to sufficient food and healthcare. How socialization affects the health of women in Bangladesh, Najma Rivzi explains in an article about a research program on this topic. In some cases, such as in parts of Kenya in 2006, rates of malnutrition in pregnant women were even higher than rates in children.

Women in some societies are traditionally given less food than men since men are perceived to have heavier workloads. Household chores and agricultural tasks can in fact be very arduous and require additional energy and nutrients; however, physical activity, which largely determines energy requirements, is difficult to estimate.

Physiology

Women have unique nutritional requirements, and in some cases need more nutrients than men; for example, women need twice as much calcium as men.

Pregnancy and Breastfeeding

During pregnancy and breastfeeding, women must ingest enough nutrients for themselves and their child, so they need significantly more protein and calories during these periods, as well as more vitamins and minerals (especially iron, iodine, calcium, folic acid, and vitamins A, C, and K). In 2001 the FAO of the UN reported that iron deficiency afflicted 43 percent of women in developing countries and increased the risk of death during childbirth. A 2008 review of interventions estimated that universal supplementation with calcium, iron, and folic acid during pregnancy could prevent 105,000 maternal deaths (23.6 percent of all maternal deaths).

Frequent pregnancies with short intervals between them and long periods of breastfeeding add an additional nutritional burden.

Educating Children

According to the FAO, women are often responsible for preparing food and have the chance to educate their children about beneficial food and health habits, giving mothers another chance to improve the nutrition of their children.

Elderly

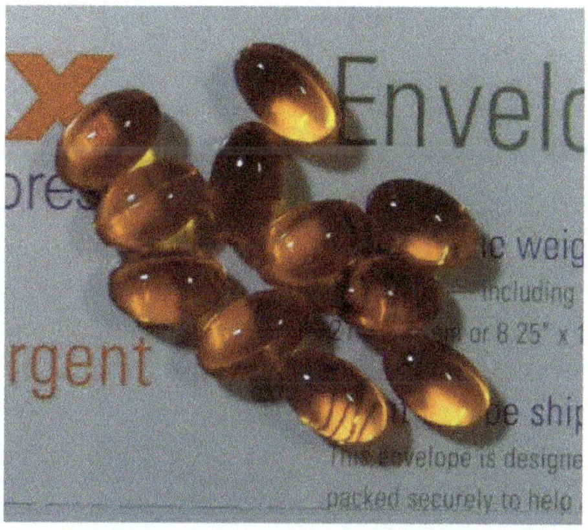

Essential nutrients are one of the main requirements of elderly care.

Malnutrition and being underweight are more common in the elderly than in adults of other ages. If elderly people are healthy and active, the aging process alone does not usually cause malnutrition. However, changes in body composition, organ functions, adequate energy intake and ability to eat or access food are associated with aging, and may contribute to malnutrition. Sadness or depression can play a role, causing changes in appetite, digestion, energy level, weight, and well-being. A study on the relationship between malnutrition and other conditions in the elderly found that Malnutrition in the elderly can result from gastrointestinal and endocrine system disorders, loss of taste and smell, decreased appetite and inadequate dietary intake. Poor dental health, ill-fitting dentures, or chewing and swallowing problems can make eating difficult. As a result of these factors, malnutrition is seen to develop more easily in the elderly.

Rates of malnutrition tend to increase with age with less than 10 percent of the "young" elderly (up to age 75) malnourished, while 30 to 65 percent of the elderly in home care, long-term care facilities, or acute hospitals are malnourished. Many elderly people require assistance in eating, which may contribute to malnutrition. Because of this, one of the main requirements of elderly care is to provide an adequate diet and all essential nutrients.

In Australia malnutrition or risk of malnutrition occurs in 80 percent of elderly people presented to hospitals for admission. Malnutrition and weight loss can contribute to sarcopenia with loss of lean body mass and muscle function. Abdominal obesity or weight loss coupled with sarcopenia lead to immobility, skeletal disorders, insulin resistance, hypertension, atherosclerosis, and metabolic disorders. A paper from the *Journal of the*

American Dietetic Association noted that routine nutrition screenings represent one way to detect and therefore decrease the prevalence of malnutrition in the elderly.

Malnutrition in Children

Malnutrition in children – here understood as undernutrition – is common globally and results in both short and long term irreversible negative health outcomes including stunted growth which may also be linked to cognitive development deficits, underweight and wasting. The World Health Organization (WHO) estimates that malnutrition accounts for 54 percent of child mortality worldwide, about 1 million children. Another estimate also by WHO states that childhood underweight is the cause for about 35% of all deaths of children under the age of five years worldwide.

The main causes are unsafe water, inadequate sanitation or insufficient hygiene, factors related to society and poverty, diseases, maternal factors, gender issues and – overall – poverty.

Signs and Symptoms

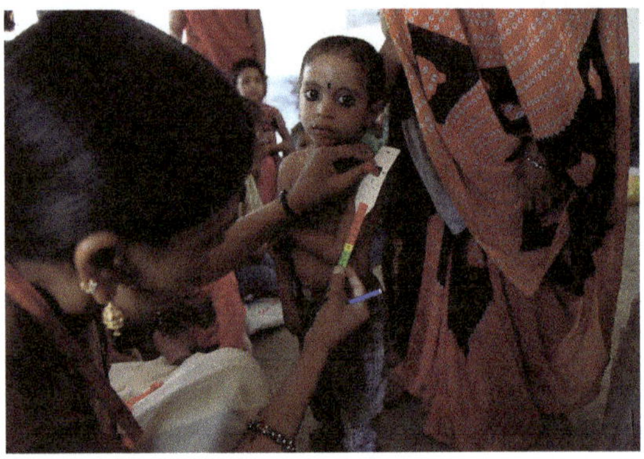

A child's upper arm is measured to detect malnutrition in the village of Baggad, in Madhya Pradesh's Dhar district (India)

Measures

There are three commonly used measures for detecting malnutrition in children:

- stunting (extremely low height for age),
- underweight (extremely low weight for age), and
- wasting (extremely low weight for height).

These measures of malnutrition are interrelated, but studies for the World Bank found that only 9 percent of children exhibit stunting, underweight, and wasting.

Children with severe acute malnutrition are very thin, but they often also have swollen hands and feet, making the internal problems more evident to health workers.

Children with severe malnutrition are very susceptible to infection.

Effects Later in Life

Undernutrition in children causes direct structural damage to the brain and impairs infant motor development and exploratory behavior. Children who are undernourished before age two and gain weight quickly later in childhood and in adolescence are at high risk of chronic diseases related to nutrition.

Studies have found a strong association between undernutrition and child mortality. Once malnutrition is treated, adequate growth is an indication of health and recovery. Even after recovering from severe malnutrition, children often remain stunted for the rest of their lives.

Even mild degrees of malnutrition double the risk of mortality for respiratory and diarrheal disease mortality and malaria. This risk is greatly increased in more severe cases of malnutrition.

Undernourished girls tend to grow into short adults and are more likely to have small children.

Prenatal malnutrition and early life growth patterns can alter metabolism and physiological patterns and have lifelong effects on the risk of cardiovascular disease. Children who are undernourished are more likely to be short in adulthood, have lower educational achievement and economic status, and give birth to smaller infants. Children often face malnutrition during the age of rapid development, which can have long-lasting impacts on health.

Causes

Inadequate food intake, infections, psychosocial deprivation, the environment (lack of sanitation and hygiene), social inequality and perhaps genetics contribute to childhood malnutrition.

Sanitation

The World Health Organisation estimated in 2008 that globally, half of all cases of undernutrition in children under five were caused by unsafe water, inadequate sanitation or insufficient hygiene. This link is often due to repeated diarrhoea and intestinal worm infections as a result of inadequate sanitation. However, the relative contribution of diarrhea to undernutrition and in turn stunting remains controversial.

Social Inequality

In almost all countries, the poorest quintile of children has the highest rate of malnutrition. However, inequalities in malnutrition between children of poor and rich families vary from country to country, with studies finding large gaps in Peru and very small gaps in Egypt. In 2000, rates of child malnutrition were much higher in low income countries (36 percent) compared to middle income countries (12 percent) and the United States (1 percent).

Studies in Bangladesh in 2009 found that the mother's literacy, low household income, higher number of siblings, less access to mass media, less supplementation of diets, unhygienic water and sanitation are associated with chronic and severe malnutrition in children.

Diseases

Diarrhea and other infections can cause malnutrition through decreased nutrient absorption, decreased intake of food, increased metabolic requirements, and direct nutrient loss. Parasite infections, in particular intestinal worm infections (helminthiasis), can also lead to malnutrition. A leading cause of diarrhea and intestinal worm infections in children in developing countries is lack of sanitation and hygiene. Other diseases that cause chronic intestinal inflammation may lead to malnutrition, such as some cases of untreated celiac disease and inflammatory bowel disease.

Children with chronic diseases like HIV have a higher risk of malnutrition, since their bodies cannot absorb nutrients as well. Diseases such as measles are a major cause of malnutrition in children; thus immunizations present a way to relieve the burden.

Maternal Factors

The nutrition of children 5 years and younger depends strongly on the nutrition level of their mothers during pregnancy and breastfeeding.

Infants born to young mothers who are not fully developed are found to have low birth weights. The level of maternal nutrition during pregnancy can affect newborn body size and composition. Iodine-deficiency in mothers usually causes brain damage in their offspring, and some cases cause extreme physical and mental retardation. This affects the children's ability to achieve their full potential. In 2011 UNICEF reported that thirty percent of households in the developing world were not consuming iodized salt, which accounted for 41 million infants and newborns in whom iodine deficiency could still be prevented. Maternal body size is strongly associated with the size of newborn children.

Short stature of the mother and poor maternal nutrition stores increase the risk of intrauterine growth retardation (IUGR). However, environmental factors can weaken the effect of IUGR on cognitive performance.

Gender

A study in Bangladesh in 2009 reported that rates of malnutrition were higher in female children than male children. Other studies show that, at the national level, differences between undernutrition prevalence rates between young boys and girls are generally small. Girls often have a lower nutritional status in South and Southeastern Asia compared to boys. In other developing regions, the nutritional status of girls is slightly higher.

Diagnosis

Measurements of a child's growth provide the key information for the presence of malnutrition, but weight and height measurements alone can lead to failure to recognize kwashiorkor and an underestimation of the severity of malnutrition in children.

Prevention

Measures have been taken to reduce child malnutrition. Studies for the World Bank found that, from 1970 to 2000, the number of malnourished children decreased by 20 percent in developing countries. Iodine supplement trials in pregnant women have been shown to reduce offspring deaths during infancy and early childhood by 29 percent. However, universal salt iodization has largely replaced this intervention.

The Progresa program in Mexico combined conditional cash transfers with nutritional education and micronutrient-fortified food supplements; this resulted in a 10 percent reduction the prevalence of stunting in children 12–36 months old. Milk fortified with zinc and iron reduced the incidence of diarrhea by 18 percent in a study in India.

Treatment

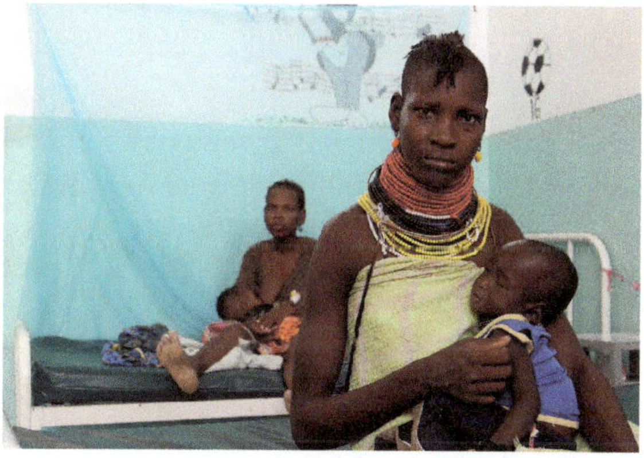

Getting support to children with malnutrition in Kenya

Treatment with antibiotics such as amoxicillin or cefdinir improve the response and survival rate of severely malnourished children to an outpatient treatment plan which provided therapeutic food. This confirms the recommendation, "In addition to the provision of RUTF [ready-to-use therapeutic food], children need to receive a short course of basic oral medication to treat infections." contained in "Community-based management of severe acute malnutrition, A Joint Statement by the World Health Organization, the World Food Programme, the United Nations System Standing Committee on Nutrition and the United Nations Children's Fund."

Breastfeeding

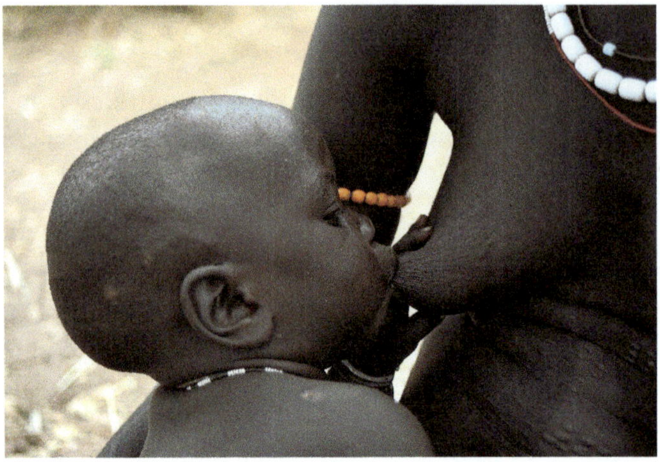

Breastfeeding can help prevent malnutrition (example from Omo Valley, Ethiopia)

Breastfeeding can reduce rates of malnutrition and dehydration caused by diarrhea, but mothers are sometimes wrongly advised to not breastfeed their children. Breastfeeding has been shown to reduce mortality in infants and young children. Since only 38 percent of children worldwide under 6 months are exclusively breastfed, education programs could have large impacts on children malnutrition rates. However, breastfeeding cannot fully prevent PEM if not enough nutrients are consumed.

Epidemiology

The World Health Organization estimates that malnutrition accounts for 54 percent of child mortality worldwide, about 1 million children. Another estimate also by WHO states that childhood underweight is the cause for about 35% of all deaths of children under the age of five years worldwide.

According to a 2008 review an estimated 178 million children under age 5 are stunted, most of whom live in sub-Saharan Africa. A 2008 review of malnutrition found that about 55 million children are wasted, including 19 million who have severe wasting or severe acute malnutrition.

As underweight children are more vulnerable to almost all infectious diseases, the *indirect* disease burden of malnutrition is estimated to be an order of magnitude higher than the disease burden of the *direct* effects of malnutrition. The combination of direct and indirect deaths from malnutrition caused by unsafe water, sanitation and hygiene (WASH) practices is estimated to lead to 860,000 deaths per year in children under five years of age.

Protein–energy Malnutrition

Protein–energy malnutrition (PEM) or protein–calorie malnutrition refers to a form of malnutrition where there is inadequate calorie or protein intake.

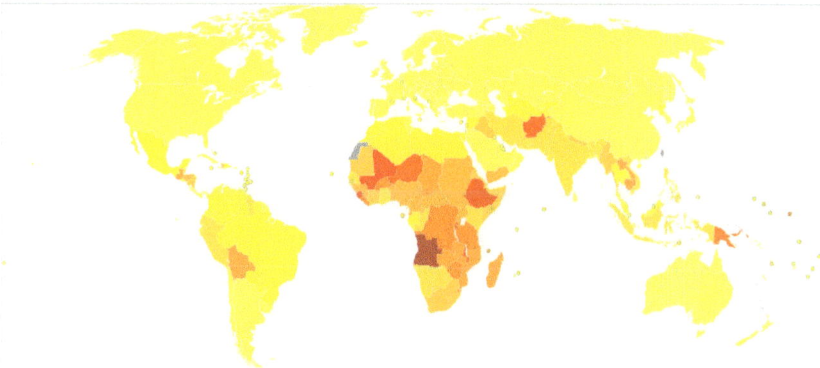

Disability-adjusted life year for protein–energy malnutrition per 100,000 inhabitants in 2004.

no data
less than 10
10–100
100–200
200–300
300–400
400–500
500–600
600–700
700–800
800–1000
1000–1350
more than 1350

Types include:

- Kwashiorkor (protein malnutrition predominant)
- Marasmus (deficiency in calorie intake)
- Marasmic Kwashiorkor (marked protein deficiency and marked calorie insufficiency signs present, sometimes referred to as the most severe form of malnutrition)

PEM is fairly common worldwide in both children and adults and accounts for 6 million deaths annually. In the industrialized world, PEM is predominantly seen in hospitals, is associated with disease, or is often found in the elderly.

Note that PEM may be secondary to other conditions such as chronic renal disease or cancer cachexia in which protein energy wasting may occur.

Protein–energy malnutrition affects children the most because they have less protein intake. The few rare cases found in the developed world are almost entirely found in small children as a result of fad diets, or ignorance of the nutritional needs of children, particularly in cases of milk allergy.

Prenatal Protein Malnutrition

Protein malnutrition is detrimental at any point in life, but protein malnutrition prenatally has been shown to have significant lifelong effects. During pregnancy, one should aim for a diet that consists of at least 20% protein for the health of the fetus. Diets that consist of less than 6% protein *in utero* have been linked with many deficits, including decreased brain weight, increased obesity, and impaired communication within the brain in some animals. Even diets of mild protein malnutrition (7.2%) have been shown to have lasting and significant effects in rats. The following are some studies in which prenatal protein deficiency has been shown to have unfavorable consequences.

- Decreased brain size: Protein deficiency has been shown to affect the size and composition of brains in rhesus monkeys. Monkeys whose mother had eaten a diet with an adequate amount of protein were shown to have no deficit in brain size or composition, even when their body weight amounted to less than one-half of that of the controls, whereas monkeys whose mothers had eaten low-protein diets were shown to have smaller brains regardless of the diet given after birth.

- Impaired neocortical long-term potentiation: Mild protein deficiency (in which 7.2% of the diet consists of protein) in rats has been shown to impair entorhinal cortex plasticity (visuospatial memory), noradrenergic function in the neocortex, and neocortical long-term potentiation.

- Altered fat distribution: Protein undernutrition can have varying effects depending on the period of fetal life during which the malnutrition occurred. Although there were not significant differences in the food intake, there were increased amounts of perirenal fat in rats that were protein-deprived during early (gestation days 0–7) and mid (gestation days 8–14) pregnancy, and throughout pregnancy, whereas rats that were protein-deprived only late in gestation (gestation days 15–22) were shown to have increased gonadal fat.

- Increased obesity: Mice exposed to a low-protein diet prenatally weighed 40% less than the control group at birth (intrauterine growth retardation). When fed a high-fat diet after birth, the prenatally undernourished mice were shown to have increased body weight and adiposity (body fat), while those who were adequately nourished prenatally did not show an increase in body weight or adiposity when fed the same high-fat diet after birth.

- Decreased birth weight, and gestation duration: Supplementation of protein and energy can lead to increased duration of gestation and higher birth weight. When fed a supplement containing protein, energy, and micronutrients, pregnant women showed more successful results during birth, including high birth weights, longer gestations, and fewer pre-term births, than women who had consumed a supplement with micronutrients and low energy but no protein (although this finding may be due to the increase of energy in the supplements, not the increase of protein).

- Increased stress sensitivity: Male offspring of pregnant rats fed low-protein diets have been shown to exhibit blood pressure that is hyperresponsive to stress and salt.

- Decreased sperm quality: A low-protein diet during gestation in rats has been shown to affect the sperm quality of the male offspring in adulthood. The protein deficiency appeared to reduce sertoli cell number, sperm motility, and sperm count.

- Altered cardiac energy metabolism: Prenatal nutrition, specifically protein nutrition, may affect the regulation of cardiac energy metabolism through changes in specific genes.

- Increased passive stiffness: Intrauterine undernutrition was shown to increase passive stiffness in skeletal muscles in rats.

From these studies it is possible to conclude that prenatal protein nutrition is vital to the development of the fetus, especially the brain, the susceptibility to diseases in adulthood, and even gene expression. When pregnant females of various species were given low-protein diets, the offspring were shown to have many deficits. These findings highlight the great significance of adequate protein in the prenatal diet.

Epidemiology

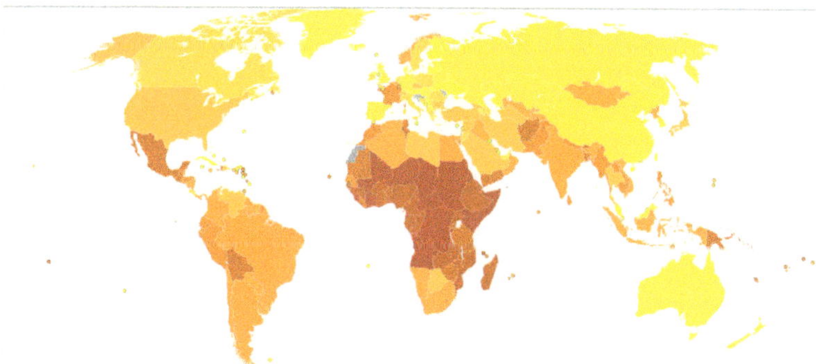

Deaths from protein-energy malnutrition per million persons in 2012

0-0	7-13	39-65
1-3	14-22	66-182
4-6	23-38	183-313
		314-923

Although protein energy malnutrition is more common in low-income countries, children from higher-income countries are also affected, including children from large urban areas in low socioeconomic neighborhoods. This may also occur in children with chronic diseases, and children who are institutionalized or hospitalized for a different diagnosis. Risk factors include a primary diagnosis of intellectual disability, cystic fibrosis, malignancy, cardiovascular disease, end stage renal disease, oncologic disease, genetic disease, neurological disease, multiple diagnoses, or prolonged hospitalization. In these conditions, the challenging nutritional management may get overlooked and underestimated, resulting in an impairment of the chances for recovery and the worsening of the situation.

PEM is fairly common worldwide in both children and adults and accounts for 6 million deaths annually. In the industrialized world, PEM is predominantly seen in hospitals, is associated with disease, or is often found in the elderly.

Co-morbidity

A large percentage of children that suffer from PEM also have other co-morbid conditions. The most common co-morbidities are diarrhea (72.2% of a sample of 66 subjects) and malaria (43.3%). However, a variety of other conditions have been observed with PEM, including sepsis, severe anaemia, bronchopneumonia, HIV, tuberculosis, scabies, chronic suppurative otitis media, rickets, and keratomalacia. These co-morbidities tax already malnourished children and may prolong hospital stays initially for PEM and may increase the likelihood of death.

Kwashiorkor

Kwashiorkor is a form of severe protein–energy malnutrition characterized by edema, irritability, ulcerating dermatoses, and an enlarged liver with fatty infiltrates. Sufficient calorie intake, but with insufficient protein consumption, distinguishes it from marasmus. Kwashiorkor cases occur in areas of famine or poor food supply. Cases in the developed world are rare.

Jamaican pediatrician Cicely Williams introduced the name into the medical community in a 1935 *Lancet* article, two years after she published the disease's first formal description in the Western medical literature. The name is derived from the Ga language of coastal Ghana, translated as "the sickness the baby gets when the new baby comes" or "the disease of the deposed child", and reflecting the development of the condition in an older child who has been weaned from the breast when a younger sibling comes. Breast milk contains proteins and amino acids vital to a child's growth. In at-risk populations, kwashiorkor may develop after a mother weans her child from breast milk, replacing it with a diet high in carbohydrates, especially sugar.

Signs and Symptoms

The defining sign of kwashiorkor in a malnourished child is pitting edema (swelling of the ankles and feet). Other signs include a distended abdomen, an enlarged liver with fatty infiltrates, thinning hair, loss of teeth, skin depigmentation and dermatitis. Children with kwashiorkor often develop irritability and anorexia. Generally, the disease can be treated by adding protein to the diet; however, it can have a long-term impact on a child's physical and mental development, and in severe cases may lead to death.

In dry climates, marasmus is the more frequent disease associated with malnutrition. Another malnutrition syndrome includes cachexia, although it is often caused by underlying illnesses. These are important considerations in the treatment of the patients.

Causes

Kwashiorkor is a severe form of malnutrition, caused by a deficiency in dietary protein. The extreme lack of protein causes an osmotic imbalance in the gastro-intestinal system causing swelling of the gut diagnosed as an edema or retention of water.

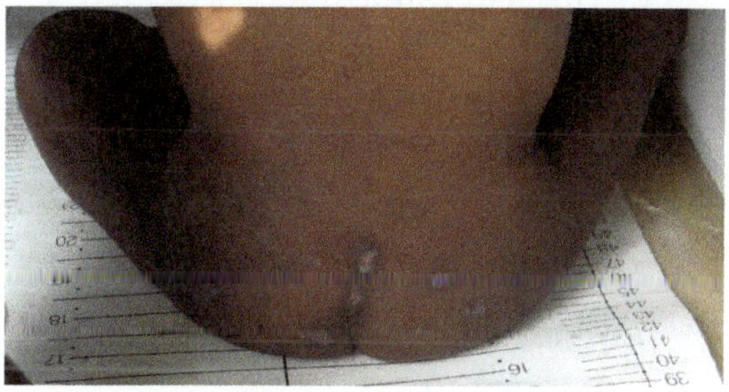

Typical ulcerating dermatosis seen on a Malawian child with kwashiorkor

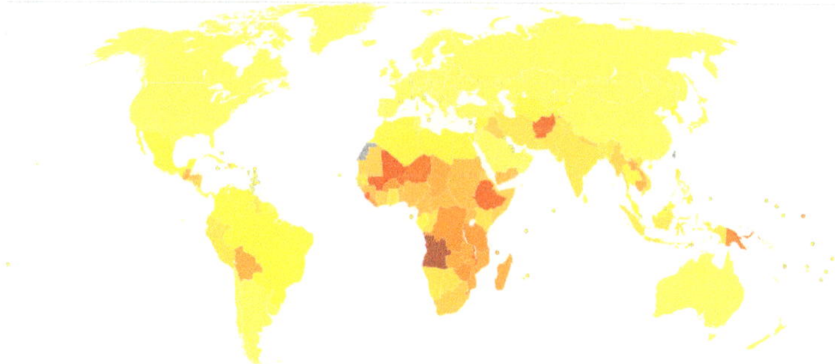

Disability-adjusted life year for protein–energy malnutrition per 100,000 inhabitants in 2002.

- no data
- fewer than 10
- 10–100
- 100–200
- 200–300
- 300–400
- 400–500
- 500–600
- 600–700
- 700–800
- 800–1000
- 1000–1350
- more than 1350

Capillary exchange between the lymphatic system and the bloodstream is stunted due to the inability of the body to effectively overcome the hydrostatic pressure gradient. Proteins, mainly albumin, are responsible for creating the colloid osmotic pressure (COP) observed in the blood and tissue fluids. The difference in the COP of the blood and tissue is called the oncotic pressure. The oncotic pressure is in direct opposition with the hydrostatic pressure and tends to draw water back into the capillary by osmosis. However, due to the lack of proteins, no substantial pressure gradient can be established to draw fluids from the tissue back into the blood stream. This results in the pooling of fluids, causing the swelling and distention of the abdomen.

The low protein intake leads to some specific signs: edema of the hands and feet, irritability, anorexia, a desquamative rash, hair discolouration, and a large fatty liver. The typical swollen abdomen is due to two causes: ascites because of hypoalbuminemia (low oncotic pressure), and enlarged fatty liver.

Ignorance of nutrition can be a cause. Dr. Michael Latham, former director of the Program in International Nutrition at Cornell University, along with Keith Rosenberg cited a case where parents who fed their child cassava failed to recognize malnutrition because of the edema caused by the syndrome and insisted the child was well-nourished despite the lack of dietary protein.

Protein should be supplied only for anabolic purposes. The catabolic needs should be satisfied with carbohydrate and fat. Protein catabolism involves the urea cycle, which is located in the liver and can easily overwhelm the capacity of an already damaged organ. The resulting liver failure can be fatal. This means in patients suffering from kwashiorkor, protein must be introduced back into the diet gradually. Clinical solutions include weaning the affected with milk products and increasing the intake of proteinaceous material to daily recommended amounts.

Prognosis

Disorders usually resolve after early treatment. If the treatment is delayed, the overall health of the child is improved but physical (reduced) and intellectual (mental disabilities) sequelae are feared. Without treatment or if treatment occurs too late, death is inevitable.

A high risk of death is identified by a brachial perimeter < 11 cm or by a weight-to-height threshold < -3 SD. In practice, malnourished children with edema are suffering from potentially life-threatening severe malnutrition.

Treatment

In order to avoid problems, the person must be rehabilitated with small but frequent rations, given every two to four hours. During one week, the diet, hyperglucidic, is gradually enriched in protein as well as essential elements: sweet milk with mineral salts and vitamins. The diet may include lactases - so that children who have developed lactose intolerance can ingest dairy products - and antibiotics - to compensate for immunodeficiency. After two to three weeks, the milk is replaced by boiled cereals fortified with minerals and vitamins until its mass is at least 80% of normal weight. Traditional food can then be reintroduced. The child is considered healed when his mass reaches 85% of normal.

Marasmus

Marasmus is a form of severe malnutrition characterized by energy deficiency. A child with marasmus looks emaciated. Body weight is reduced to less than 62.36% of the normal (expected) body weight for the age. Marasmus occurrence increases prior to age 1, whereas kwashiorkor occurrence increases after 18 months. It can be distinguished from kwashiorkor in that kwashiorkor is protein deficiency with adequate energy intake whereas marasmus is inadequate energy intake in all forms, including protein. This clear-cut separation of marasmus and kwashiorkor is however not always clinically evident as kwashiorkor is often seen in a context of insufficient caloric intake, and mixed clinical pictures, called marasmic kwashiorkor, are possible. Protein wasting in kwashiorkor generally leads to edema and ascites, while muscular wasting and loss of subcutaneous fat are the main clinical signs of marasmus.

The prognosis is better than it is for kwashiorkor but half of severely malnourished children die due to unavailability of adequate treatment.

The word "marasmus" comes from the Greek *marasmos* ("withering").

Signs and Symptoms

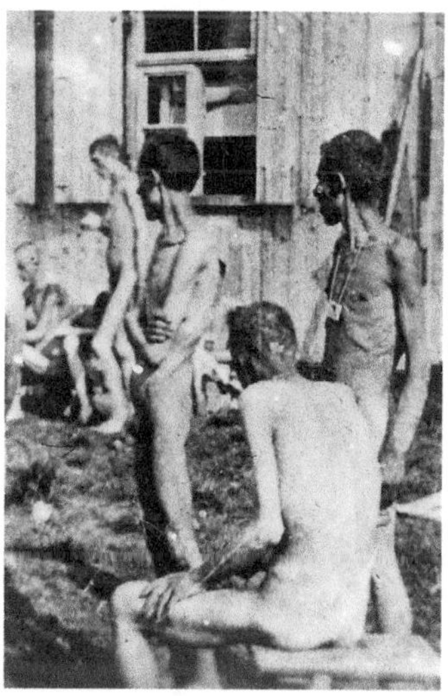

Buchenwald inmates, 16 April 1945 when camp was liberated

Marasmus is commonly represented by a shrunken, wasted appearance, loss of muscle mass and subcutaneous fat mass. Buttocks and upper limb muscle groups are usually more affected than others. Edema is not a sign of marasmus and is only present in kwashiorkor, and marasmic kwashiorkor. Other symptoms of marasmus include unusual body temperature (hypothermia, pyrexia), anemia, dehydration (as characterized with consistent thirst and shrunken eyes), hypovolemic shock (weak radial pulse, cold extremities, decreased consciousness), tachypnea (pneumonia, heart failure), abdominal manifestations (distension, decreased or metallic bowel sounds, large or small liver, blood or mucus in the stools), ocular manifestations (corneal lesions associated with vitamin A deficiency), dermal manifestations (evidence of infection, purpura, and ear, nose, and throat symptoms (otitis, rhinitis).

Causes

Marasmus is caused by a severe deficiency of nearly all nutrients, especially protein, carbohydrates, and lipids.

Viral, bacterial, and parasitic infections can cause children to take in too few nutrients. Marasmus can develop in children who suffer from weakening conditions such as chronic diarrhea.

Treatment

It is necessary to treat not only the causes but also the complications of the disorder, including infections, dehydration, and circulation disorders, which are frequently lethal and lead to high mortality if ignored.

Ultimately, marasmus can progress to the point of no return when the body's ability for protein synthesis is lost. At this point, attempts to correct the disorder by giving food or protein are futile.

Epidemiology

Persons in prisons, concentration camps, and refugee camps tend to suffer from marasmus, due to poor nutrition.

Catabolysis

Catabolysis is a biological process in which the body breaks down fat and muscle tissue in order to stay alive. Catabolysis occurs only when there is no longer any source of protein, carbohydrate, or vitamin nourishment feeding all body systems; it is the most severe type of malnutrition.

Mechanism

Due to the normal metabolic rate of humans catabolysis becomes life-threatening only after 1–2 months from the cessation of nutrition going into the body. After this time, the damage to muscles and organs can be permanent and can also eventually cause death, if left untreated. Catabolysis is the last metabolic resort for the body to keep itself – particularly the nervous system—functional.

Protein stores, especially in muscle tissue, provide the amino acids needed for the process. Amino acids are released into the blood and converted in the liver to alpha keto acids. Alpha keto acids can then be converted to glucose to maintain proper blood sugar levels.

The situation can become dire when one begins to lose muscle mass; this is a sign that the fat has been expended and the body is now metabolizing the muscle tissue. This results in muscle atrophy, a loss of strength and, ultimately, a depletion of muscular tissue completely. Muscle weakness is not necessarily a symptom of catabolysis: the muscles will normally feel fatigued when they are not receiving enough energy or oxygen. Ultimately, catabolysis can progress to the point of no return when the body's machinery for protein synthesis, itself made of protein, has been degraded to the point that it cannot handle any protein. At this point, attempts to correct the disorder by giving food or protein are futile.

The body has a natural store of fat (also called *adipose tissue*) that stores reserve energy. One can still stay alive while the body breaks down the fatty tissue (hence people wasting away from starvation).

The person may, during catabolysis, have large amounts of lipids, proteins, and amino acids in the bloodstream, due to the muscle fibers and adipose tissues being broken down and sent to the nervous system and brain. One may also exhibit a fever, since the body is working hard to transfer the nutrients in the muscles and fat to the blood.

Treatment

While catabolysis can be deadly over time, if the person is given medical treatment early enough, the effects of catabolysis can be reversed. However, the person may require intravenous nutrition, a blood transfusion, and/or oxygen replenishment. After that, it may be a few weeks to a few months before the person's muscle mass and fat deposits can build themselves up again; there is a possibility that they may never build back up, depending on the severity of the condition.

Protein Poisoning

Protein poisoning (also referred to colloquially as rabbit starvation, *mal de caribou*, or fat starvation) is a rare form of acute malnutrition thought to be caused by a complete absence of fat in the diet.

Excess protein is sometimes cited as the cause of this issue; when meat and fat are consumed in the correct ratio, such as that found in pemmican (which is 50% fat by volume), the diet is considered nutritionally complete and can support humans for months or more. Other stressors, such as severe cold or a dry environment, may intensify symptoms or decrease time to onset. Symptoms include diarrhea, headache, fatigue, low blood pressure, slow heart rate, and a vague discomfort and hunger (very similar to a food craving) that can be satisfied only by the consumption of fat.

Protein poisoning was first noted as a consequence of eating rabbit meat exclusively, hence the term, "rabbit starvation". Rabbit meat is very lean; commercial rabbit meat has 50–100 g dissectable fat per 2 kg (live weight). Based on a carcass yield of 60%, rabbit meat is around 8.3% fat. For comparison, in terms of carcass composition, beef and pork are 32% fat and lamb 28%.

Possible Mechanisms

It has been observed that the human liver cannot safely metabolise much more than 221–301 g of protein per day (for an 80 kg/176 pound person), and human kidneys are similarly limited in their capability to remove urea (a byproduct of protein catabolism) from the bloodstream. Exceeding that amount results in excess levels of amino acids, ammonia (hyperammonemia), and/or urea in the bloodstream, with potentially fatal consequences, especially if the person switches to a high-protein diet without giving time for the levels of his or her hepatic enzymes to upregulate. Since protein only contains 4 kcal/gram, and a typical adult human requires in excess of 1900 kcal to maintain the energy balance, it is possible to exceed the safe intake of protein if one is subjected to a high-protein diet with little or no fat or carbohydrates. However, given the lack of scientific data on the effects of high-protein diets, and the observed ability of the liver to compensate over a few days for a shift in protein intake, the US Food and Nutrition Board does not set a tolerable upper intake level nor upper acceptable macronutrient distribution range for protein.

Observations

The Arctic explorer Vilhjalmur Stefansson wrote as follows:

The groups that depend on the blubber animals are the most fortunate in the hunting way of life, for they never suffer from fat-hunger. This trouble is worst, so far as North America is concerned, among those forest Indians who depend at times on rabbits, the leanest animal in the North, and who develop the extreme fat-hunger known as rabbit-starvation. Rabbit eaters, if they have no fat from another source—beaver, moose, fish—will develop diarrhea in about a week, with headache, lassitude and vague discomfort. If there are enough rabbits, the people eat till their stomachs are distended; but no matter how much they eat they feel unsatisfied. Some think a man will die sooner if he eats continually of fat-free meat than if he eats nothing, but this is a belief on which sufficient evidence for a decision has not been gathered in the North. Deaths from rabbit-starvation, or from the eating of other skinny meat, are rare; for everyone understands the principle, and any possible preventive steps are naturally taken.

During the Greely Arctic Expedition 1881–1884, a harrowing experience of 25 expedition members, of whom 19 died, Stefansson refers to "'rabbit starvation' which is now to me the key to the Greely problem," which was why "only six came back." He concludes that one of the reasons for the many deaths was cannibalism of the lean flesh of members who had already died. Stefansson likens this to rabbit starvation, which he explains somewhat as in the above quoted observation.

Charles Darwin, in *The Voyage of the Beagle*, wrote:

We were here able to buy some biscuit. I had now been several days without tasting any thing besides meat: I did not at all dislike this new regimen; but I felt as if it would only have agreed with me with hard exercise. I have heard that patients in England, when desired to confine themselves exclusively to an animal diet, even with the hope of life before their eyes, have hardly been able to endure it. Yet the Gaucho in the Pampas, for months together, touches nothing but beef. But they eat, I observe, a very large proportion of fat, which is of a less animalized nature; and they particularly dislike dry meat, such as that of the Agouti. Dr. Richardson, also, has remarked, "that when people have fed for a long time solely upon lean animal food, the desire for fat becomes so insatiable, that they can consume a large quantity of unmixed and even oily fat without nausea:" this appears to me a curious physiological fact. It is, perhaps, from their meat regimen that the Gauchos, like other carnivorous animals, can abstain long from food. I was told that at Tandeel, some troops voluntarily pursued a party of Indians for three days, without eating or drinking.

In *Into the Wild* (1996), Jon Krakauer conjectured that Chris McCandless might have suffered from rabbit starvation.

Malabsorption

Malabsorption is a state arising from abnormality in absorption of food nutrients across the gastrointestinal (GI) tract. Impairment can be of single or multiple nutrients depending on the abnormality. This may lead to malnutrition and a variety of anaemias.

Normally the human gastrointestinal tract digests and absorbs dietary nutrients with remarkable efficiency. A typical Western diet ingested by an adult includes approximately 100 g of fat, 400 g of carbohydrate, 100 g of protein, 2 L of fluid, and the required sodium, potassium, chloride, calcium, vitamins, and other elements. Salivary, gastric, intestinal, hepatic, and pancreatic secretions add an additional 7–8 L of protein-, lipid-, and electrolyte-containing fluid to intestinal contents. This massive load is reduced by the small and large intestines to less than 200 g of stool that contains less than 8 g of fat, 1–2 g of nitrogen, and less than 20 mmol each of Na^+, K^+, Cl^-, HCO_3^-, Ca^{2+}, or Mg^{2+}.

If there is impairment of any of the many steps involved in the complex process of nutrient digestion and absorption, intestinal *malabsorption* may ensue. If the abnormality involves a single step in the absorptive process, as in primary lactase deficiency, or if the disease process is limited to the very proximal small intestine selective malabsorption of only a single nutrient may occur. However, generalized *malabsorption* of multiple dietary nutrients develops when the disease process is extensive, thus disturbing several digestive and absorptive processes, as occurs in coeliac disease with extensive involvement of the small intestine.

Classification

Some prefer to classify malabsorption clinically into three basic categories:

1. selective, as seen in lactose malabsorption.
2. partial, as observed in abetalipoproteinaemia.
3. total, as in exceptional cases of coeliac disease.

Signs and Symptoms

Gastrointestinal Manifestations

Depending on the nature of the disease process causing malabsorption and its extent, gastrointestinal symptoms may range from severe to subtle or may even be totally absent. Diarrhea, weight loss, flatulence, abdominal bloating, abdominal cramps, and pain may be present. Although diarrhea is a common complaint, the character and frequency of stools may vary considerably ranging from over 10 watery stools per day to less than one voluminous putty-like stool, the latter causing some patients to complain of constipation. On the other hand, stool mass is invariably increased in patients with steatorrhea and generalized malabsorption above the normal with 150–200 g/day. Not only do unabsorbed nutrients contribute to stool mass but mucosal fluid and electrolyte secretion is also increased in diseases associated with mucosal inflammation such as coeliac disease. In addition, unabsorbed fatty acids, converted to hydroxy-fatty acids by colonic flora, as well as unabsorbed bile acids both impair absorption and induce secretion of water and electrolytes by the colon adding to stool mass. Weight loss is common among patients with significant intestinal malabsorption but must be evaluated in the context of caloric intake. Some patients compensate for fecal wastage of unabsorbed nutrients by significantly increasing their oral intake. Eliciting a careful dietary history from patients with suspected malabsorption is therefore crucial. Excessive flatus and abdominal bloating may reflect excessive gas production due to fermentation of unabsorbed carbohydrate, especially among patients with primary or secondary disaccharidase deficiency. Malabsorption of dietary nutrients and excessive fluid secretion by inflamed small intestine also contribute to abdominal distention and bloating. Prevalence, severity, and character of abdominal pain vary considerably among the various disease processes associated with intestinal malabsorption. For example, pain is common in patients with chronic pancreatitis or pancreatic cancer and Crohn disease, but it is absent in many patients with coeliac disease or postgastrectomy malabsorption.

Extraintestinal Manifestations

Substantial numbers of patients with intestinal malabsorption present initially with symptoms or laboratory abnormalities that point to other organ systems in the absence of or overshadowing symptoms referable to the gastrointestinal tract. For example, there is increasing epidemiologic evidence that more patients with coeliac disease present with anemia and osteopenia in the absence of significant classic gastrointestinal symptoms. Microcytic, macrocytic, or dimorphic anemia may reflect impaired iron, folate, or vitamin B12 absorption. Purpura, subconjunctival hemorrhage, or even frank bleeding may reflect hypoprothrombinemia secondary to vitamin K malabsorption. Osteopenia is common, especially in the presence of steatorrhea. Impaired calcium and vitamin D absorption and chelation of calcium by unabsorbed fatty acids resulting in fecal loss of calcium may all contribute. If calcium deficiency is prolonged, secondary hyperparathyroidism may develop. Prolonged malnutrition may induce amenorrhea, infertility, and impotence. Edema and even ascites may reflect hypoproteinemia associated with protein losing enteropathy caused by lymphatic obstruction or extensive mucosal inflammation. Dermatitis and peripheral neuropathy may be caused by malabsorption of specific vitamins or micronutrients and essential fatty acids.

Pathophysiology

The main purpose of the gastrointestinal tract is to digest and absorb nutrients (fat, carbohydrate, protein, micronutrients (vitamins and trace minerals), water, and electrolytes. Digestion involves both mechanical and enzymatic breakdown of food. Mechanical processes include chewing, gastric churning, and the to-and-fro mixing in the small intestine. Enzymatic hydrolysis is initiated by intraluminal processes requiring gastric, pancreatic, and biliary secretions. The final products of digestion are absorbed through the intestinal epithelial cells.

Malabsorption constitutes the pathological interference with the normal physiological sequence of digestion (intraluminal process), absorption (mucosal process) and transport (postmucosal events) of nutrients.

Intestinal malabsorption can be due to:

- Mucosal damage (enteropathy)
- Congenital or acquired reduction in absorptive surface
- Defects of specific hydrolysis
- Defects of ion transport
- Pancreatic insufficiency
- Impaired enterohepatic circulation

Causes

Due to infective agents

- HIV related malabsorption
- Traveler's diarrhea
- Parasites e.g. *Giardia lamblia*, fish tape worm (B_{12} malabsorption); roundworm, hookworm (*Ancylostoma duodenale* and *Necator americanus*)
- Tropical sprue
- Whipple's disease
- Intestinal tuberculosis

Due to structural defects

- Blind loops
- Inflammatory bowel diseases, as in Crohn's Disease
- Fistulae, diverticula and strictures
- Infiltrative conditions such as amyloidosis, lymphoma, eosinophilic gastro-enteritis
- Radiation enteritis
- Systemic sclerosis and collagen vascular diseases
- Short bowel syndrome

Due to surgical structural changes

- Gastrectomy; Vagotomy
- Bariatric surgery (Weight loss surgery)

Due to mucosal abnormality

- Coeliac disease
- Cows' milk intolerance
- Soya milk intolerance
- Fructose malabsorption

Due to enzyme deficiencies

- Lactase deficiency inducing lactose intolerance (constitutional, secondary or rarely congenital)

- Sucrose intolerance
- Intestinal disaccharidase deficiency
- Intestinal enteropeptidase deficiency

Due to digestive failure

- Pancreatic insufficiencies:
  - o Cystic fibrosis
  - o Chronic pancreatitis
  - o Carcinoma of pancreas
- Zollinger-Ellison syndrome
- Bile acid/Bile salt malabsorption
  - o Terminal ileal disease such as Crohn's disease
  - o Obstructive jaundice
  - o Bacterial overgrowth
  - o Primary bile acid diarrhea

Clinical Features

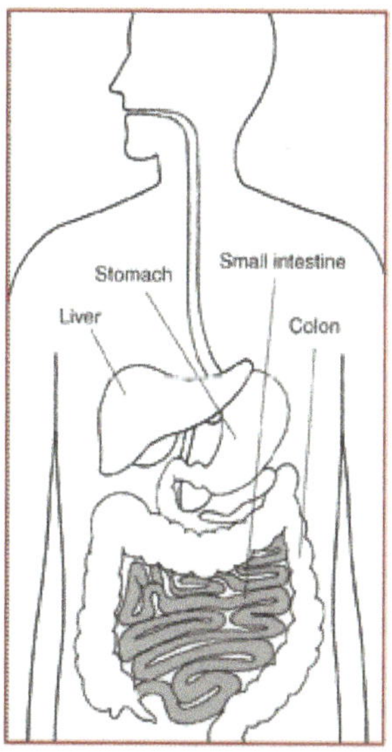

Small intestine : major site of absorption

They can occur in a variety of ways and features might give a clue to the underlying condition. Symptoms can be intestinal or extra-intestinal - the former predominates in severe malabsorption.

- Diarrhoea, often steatorrhoea, is the most common feature. Watery, diurnal and nocturnal, bulky, frequent stools are the clinical hallmark of overt malabsorption. It is due to impaired water, carbohydrate and electrolyte absorption or irritation from unabsorbed fatty acid. The latter also results in bloating, flatulence and abdominal discomfort. Cramping pain usually suggests obstructive intestinal segment e.g. in Crohn's disease, especially if it persists after defecation.
- Weight loss can be significant despite increased oral intake of nutrients.
- Growth retardation, failure to thrive, delayed puberty in children
- Swelling or oedema from loss of protein
- Anaemias, commonly from vitamin B_{12}, folic acid and iron deficiency presenting as fatigue and weakness.
- Muscle cramp from decreased vitamin D, calcium absorption. Also lead to osteomalacia and osteoporosis
- Bleeding tendencies from vitamin K and other coagulation factor deficiencies.

Diagnosis

There is no single, specific test for malabsorption. As for most medical conditions, investigation is guided by symptoms and signs. A range of different conditions can produce malabsorption and it is necessary to look for each of these specifically. Many tests have been advocated, and some, such as tests for pancreatic function are complex, vary between centers and have not been widely adopted. However, better tests have become available with greater ease of use, better sensitivity and specificity for the causative conditions. Tests are also needed to detect the systemic effects of deficiency of the malabsorbed nutrients (such as anaemia with vitamin B12 malabsorption).

Blood Tests

- Routine blood tests may reveal anaemia, high CRP or low albumin; which shows a high correlation for the presence of an organic disease. In this setting, microcytic anaemia usually implies iron deficiency and macrocytosis can be caused by impaired folic acid or B12 absorption or both. Low cholesterol or triglyceride may give a clue toward fat malabsorption. Low calcium and phosphate may give a clue toward osteomalacia from low vitamin D.
- Specific vitamins like vitamin D or micro nutrient like zinc levels can be checked. Fat soluble vitamins (A, D, E & K) are affected in fat malabsorption. Prolonged prothrombin time can be caused by vitamin K deficiency.
- Serological studies. Specific tests are carried out to determine the underlying cause.

IgA Anti-transglutaminase antibodies or IgA Anti-endomysial antibodies for Coeliac disease (gluten sensitive enteropathy).

Stool Studies

- Microscopy is particularly useful in diarrhoea, may show protozoa like Giardia, ova, cyst and other infective agents.
- Fecal fat study to diagnose steatorrhoea is rarely performed nowadays.
- Low fecal pancreatic elastase is indicative of pancreatic insufficiency. Chymotrypsin and pancreolauryl can be assessed as well

Radiological Studies

- Barium follow through is useful in delineating small intestinal anatomy. Barium enema may be undertaken to see colonic or ileal lesions.
- CT abdomen is useful in ruling out structural abnormality, done in pancreatic protocol when visualising pancreas.
- Magnetic resonance cholangiopancreatography (MRCP) to complement or as an alternative to ERCP.

Interventional Studies

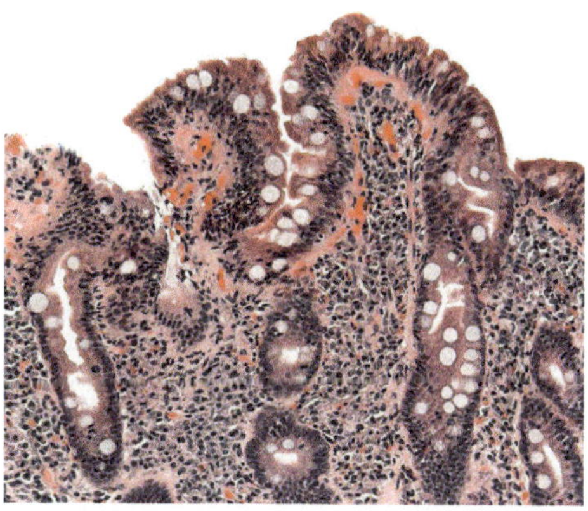

Biopsy of small bowel showing coeliac disease manifested by blunting of villi, crypt hyperplasia, and lymphocyte infiltration of crypts.

- OGD to detect duodenal pathology and obtain D2 biopsy (for coeliac disease, tropical sprue, Whipple's disease, abetalipoproteinaemia etc.)
- Enteroscopy for enteropathy and jejunal aspirate and culture for bacterial overgrowth
- Capsule Endoscopy is able to visualise the whole small intestine and is occasionally useful.

- Colonoscopy is necessary in colonic and ileal disease.
- ERCP will show pancreatic and biliary structural abnormalities.

Other Investigations

- 75SeHCAT test to diagnose bile acid malabsorption in ileal disease or primary bile acid diarrhea.
- Glucose hydrogen breath test for bacterial overgrowth
- Lactose hydrogen breath test for lactose intolerance
- Sugar probes or ^{51}Cr-EDTA to determine intestinal permeability.

Obsolete Tests no Longer used Clinically

- D-xylose absorption test for mucosal disease or bacterial overgrowth. Normal in pancreatic insufficiency.
- Bile salt breath test (^{14}C-glycocholate) to determine bile salt malabsorption.
- Schilling test to establish cause of B_{12} deficiency.

Management

Treatment is directed largely towards management of underlying cause:

- Replacement of nutrients, electrolytes and fluid may be necessary. In severe deficiency, hospital admission may be required for nutritional support and detailed advice from dietitians. Use of enteral nutrition by naso-gastric or other feeding tubes may be able to provide sufficient nutritional supplementation. Tube placement may also be done by percutaneous endoscopic gastrostomy, or surgical jejunostomy. In patients whose intestinal absorptive surface is severely limited from disease or surgery, long term total parenteral nutrition may be needed.
- Pancreatic enzymes are supplemented orally in pancreatic insufficiency.
- Dietary modification is important in some conditions:
    - o Gluten-free diet in coeliac disease.
    - o Lactose avoidance in lactose intolerance.
- Antibiotic therapy to treat Small Bowel Bacterial overgrowth.
- Cholestyramine or other bile acid sequestrants will help reducing diarrhoea in bile acid malabsorption.

References

- Parham, Peter (20 May 2014). The Immune System. New York: Garland Science Taylor and Francis Group LLC. p. 494. ISBN 978-0-8153-4146-8
- Nubé, M.; Van Den Boom, G. J. M. (2003). "Gender and adult undernutrition in developing countries". Annals of Human Biology. 30 (5): 520–537. PMID 12959894. doi:10.1080/0301446031000119601
- Rasmussen KM, Habicht JP (February 2010). "Maternal supplementation differentially affects the mother and newborn". The Journal of Nutrition. 140 (2): 402–6. PMID 20032480. doi:10.3945/jn.109.114488
- Walker, [edited by] Christopher Duggan, John B. Watkins, W. Allan (2008). Nutrition in pediatrics: basic science, clinical application. Hamilton: BC Decker. pp. 127–141. ISBN 978-1-55009-361-2
- Sue Horton; Harold Alderman, Juan A. Rivera (2008). "The Challenge of Hunger and Malnutrition" (PDF). Copenhagen Consensus Challenge Paper. Archived from the original (PDF) on November 15, 2012. Retrieved March 3, 2014
- Bosaeus, Ingvar (2008). "Nutritional support in multimodal therapy for cancer cachexia". Supportive Care in Cancer. 16 (5): 447–51. PMID 18196284. doi:10.1007/s00520-007-0388-7
- Bilsborough, S.; Mann, N. (April 2006). "A review of issues of dietary protein intake in humans". International Journal of Sport Nutrition and Exercise Metabolism. 16 (2): 129–152. PMID 16779921
- World Bank (2008). Environmental health and child survival epidemiology, economics, experiences. Washington, DC: Environment Department of the World Bank. ISBN 978-0-8213-7237-1
- Jakoby, WB; Ziegler, DM (5 December 1990). "The enzymes of detoxication.". The Journal of biological chemistry. 265 (34): 20715–8. PMID 2249981
- Ruppert EE, Fox RS, Barnes RD (2004). "Introduction to Eumetazoa". Invertebrate Zoology (7 ed.). Brooks / Cole. pp. 99–103. ISBN 0-03-025982-7
- Jensen, Jonathan E. "Malabsorption Syndromes - Page 1". Colorado center for digestive disorders. Archived from the original on 2007-04-11. Retrieved 2007-05-10
- Tipton, K (May 2011). "Efficacy and consequences of very-high-protein diets for athletes and exercisers.". Proceedings of the Nutrition Society. 70 (2): 205–14. PMID 21375795. doi:10.1017/S0029665111000024
- Fox, James; Timothy Wang (January 2007). "Inflammation, Atrophy, and Gastric Cancer". Journal of Clinical Investigation. review. 117 (1): 60–69. PMC 1716216 . PMID 17200707. doi:10.1172/JCI30111. Retrieved 19 May 2014
- Abraham L. Kierszenbaum (2002). Histology and cell biology: an introduction to pathology. St. Louis: Mosby. ISBN 0-323-01639-1
- Kapoor, Vinay Kumar (13 Jul 2011). Gest, Thomas R., ed. "Large Intestine Anatomy". Medscape. WebMD LLC. Retrieved 2013-08-20
- Newnham ED (2017). "Coeliac disease in the 21st century: paradigm shifts in the modern age.". J Gastroenterol Hepatol (Review). 32 Suppl 1: 82–85. PMID 28244672. doi:10.1111/jgh.13704

2

Overnutrition: An Integrated Study

Overnutrition is caused by excessive intake of nutrients. Excess of nutrients can lead to iron poisoning. Being overweight and hypervitaminosis are some complications related to overnutrition. The topics elaborated in this chapter will help in gaining a better perspective about the concept of overnutrition.

Overnutrition

Overnutrition or hyperalimentation is a form of malnutrition in which the intake of nutrients is oversupplied. The amount of nutrients exceeds the amount required for normal growth, development, and metabolism.

The term can also refer to:

- Obesity, which *usually* occurs by overeating, as well as:
- Oversupplying a *specific* nutrient, such as dietary minerals or vitamin poisoning. This is due to an excessive intake or a nutritional imbalance caused by fad diets.

For mineral excess:

- Iron poisoning, and
- Low sodium diet (a response to excess sodium).

Overnutrition may also refers to greater food consumption than appropriate, as well as other feeding procedures such as parenteral nutrition.

Iron Poisoning

Iron poisoning is an iron overload caused by a large excess of iron intake and usually refers to an acute overload rather than a gradual one. The term has been primarily associated with young children who consumed large quantities of iron supplement pills, which resemble sweets and are widely used, including by pregnant women; approximately 3 grams is lethal for a two-year-old. Targeted packaging restrictions in the US for supplement containers with over 250 mg elemental iron have existed since 1978, and recommendations for unit packaging have reduced the several iron poisoning fatalities per year to almost zero since 1998. No known cases of iron poisoning have been identified that are associated with iron mining.

Signs and Symptoms

The first indication of iron poisoning by ingestion is stomach pain, as iron is corrosive to the lining of the gastrointestinal tract, including the stomach. Nausea and vomiting are also common symptoms and bloody vomiting may occur. The pain then abates for 24 hours as the iron passes deeper into the body, resulting in metabolic acidosis, which in turn damages internal organs, particularly the brain and the liver. Iron poisoning can cause hypovolemic shock due to iron's potent ability to dilate the blood vessels. Death may occur from liver failure.

If intake of iron is for a prolonged period of time, symptoms are likely to be similar to other causes of iron overload.

Cause

In nature, iron is usually found in its oxidized form, iron (III) oxide, which is insoluble. Ferrous iron, iron (II), is soluble and its toxicity varies, largely with the integrity of the gastrointestinal lining. Iron supplements are typically used to treat anemia. Modalities include: diet, parasite control, vitamin A, riboflavin (B_2), vitamin C (for absorption), folate(B_9), vitamin B_{12} and multivitamin-multimineral supplements, with or without iron; potentially avoiding the use of iron only supplements.

Toxic Dose

The amount of iron ingested may give a clue to potential toxicity. The therapeutic dose for iron deficiency anemia is 3–6 mg/kg/day. Toxic effects begin to occur at doses above 10–20 mg/kg of elemental iron. Ingestions of more than 50 mg/kg of elemental iron are associated with severe toxicity.

- A 325-mg tablet of ferrous sulfate heptahydrate has 65 mg (20%) of elemental iron
- A 325-mg tablet of ferrous gluconate has 39 mg (12%) of elemental iron
- A 325-mg tablet of ferrous fumarate has 107.25 mg (33%) of elemental iron
- 200 mg ferrous sulfate, dried, has 65 mg (33%) of elemental iron

In terms of blood values, iron levels above 350–500 µg/dL are considered toxic, and levels over 1000 µg/dL indicate severe iron poisoning.

Treatment

Later stage treatment consists of cleaning the iron from the blood, using a chelating agent such as deferoxamine. If this fails then dialysis is the next step.

Calorie Restriction

Calorie restriction, or caloric restriction, or energy restriction, is a dietary regimen that reduces calorie intake without incurring malnutrition or a reduction in essential nutrients. "Low" can be defined relative to the subject's previous intake before intentionally restricting calories, or relative to an average person of similar body type. In a number of species, including yeast, fish, rodents and dogs, calorie restriction without malnutrition has been shown to slow the biological aging process, resulting in longer maintenance of youthful health and an increase in both median and maximum lifespan. However, the life-extending effect of calorie restriction is not shown to be universal.

In humans, the long-term health effects of moderate caloric restriction with sufficient nutrients are unknown.

Using rhesus monkeys – which harbor 93% of the human genome – a collaboration of the United States National Institute on Aging and the University of Wisconsin found that caloric restriction without malnutrition extended lifespan and delayed the onset of age-related disorders; older age, higher diet quality, and female gender were positive factors affecting the benefits realized from lower caloric intake.

Health Effects

In humans the long-term health effects of moderate caloric restriction with sufficient nutrients are unknown.

Risks of Malnutrition

As noted above, the term "calorie restriction" as used in biogerontology refers to dietary regimens that reduce calorie intake without incurring malnutrition. If a restricted diet is not designed to include essential nutrients, malnutrition may result in serious deleterious effects, as shown in the Minnesota Starvation Experiment. This study was conducted during World War II on a group of lean men, who restricted their calorie intake by 45% for 6 months, and composed roughly 90% of their diet with carbohydrates. As expected, this malnutrition resulted in many positive metabolic adaptations (e.g. decreased body fat, blood pressure, improved lipid profile, low serum T3 concentration, and decreased resting heart rate and whole-body resting energy expenditure), but also caused a wide range of negative effects, such as anemia, lower extremity edema, muscle wasting, weakness, neurological deficits, dizziness, irritability, lethargy, and depression.

Musculoskeletal Losses

Short-term studies in humans report loss of muscle mass and strength and reduced bone mineral density. However, whether or not the reduction in bone mineral density actually harms bone health is unclear. In a study in premenopausal women, bone mineral density after weight loss was higher when normalized for body weight; reduced bone mineral density is also observed in humans undergoing long-term calorie restriction with adequate nutrition, but no fractures have been reported and the reduction in bone mineral density was not associated with deleterious changes in bone microarchitecture.

The authors of a 2007 review of the caloric restriction literature warned that "[i]t is possible that even moderate calorie restriction may be harmful in specific patient populations, such as lean persons who have minimal amounts of body fat."

Lower-than-normal Body Mass Index, High Mortality

Caloric restriction diets typically lead to reduced body weight, yet reduced weight can come from other causes and is not in itself necessarily healthy. In some studies, low body weight has been associated with increased mortality, particularly in late middle-aged or elderly subjects. Low body weight in the elderly can be caused by pathological conditions associated with aging and predisposing to higher mortality (such as cancer, chronic obstructive pulmonary disorder, or depression) or of the cachexia (wasting syndrome) and sarcopenia (loss of muscle mass, structure, and function). One of the more famous of such studies linked a body mass index lower than 18 in women with increased mortality from noncancer, non–cardiovascular disease causes. The authors attempted to adjust for confounding factors (cigarette smoking, failure to exclude pre-existing disease); others argued that the adjustments were inadequate.

> "epidemiologists from the ACS (American Cancer Society), American Heart Association, Harvard School of Public Health, and other organizations raised specific methodologic questions about the recent Centers for Disease Control and Prevention study and presented analyses of other data sets. The main concern ... is that it did not adequately account for weight loss from serious illnesses such as cancer and heart disease ... [and] failed to account adequately for the effect of smoking on weight ... As a result, the Flegal study underestimated the risks from obesity and overestimated the risks of leanness."

Such epidemiological studies of body weight are not about caloric restriction as used in anti-aging studies; they are not about caloric intake to begin with, as body weight is influenced by many factors other than energy intake. Moreover, "the quality of the diets consumed by the low-body mass index individuals are difficult to assess, and may lack nutrients important to longevity." Typical low-calorie diets rarely provide the high nutrient intakes that are a necessary feature of an anti-aging calorie restriction diet. As well, "The lower-weight individuals in the studies are not caloric restriction because their caloric intake reflects their individual ad libitum set-points, and not a reduction from that set-point."

Triggering Binge Eating

In those who already suffer from a binge-eating disorder, calorie restriction can precipitate an episode of binge eating, but it does not seem to pose any such risk otherwise.

Young or Pregnant

Long-term caloric restriction at a level sufficient for slowing the aging process is generally not recommended in children, adolescents, and young adults (under the age of approximately 21), because this type of diet may interfere with natural physical growth, as has been observed in laboratory animals. In addition, mental development and physical changes to the brain take place in late adolescence and early adulthood that could be negatively affected by severe caloric restriction. Pregnant women and women trying to become pregnant are advised not to practice calorie restriction, because low BMI may result in ovulatory dysfunction (infertility), and underweight mothers are more prone to preterm delivery.

Miscellaneous Concerns

It has also been noted that people losing weight on such diets risk developing cold sensitivity, menstrual irregularities, and even infertility and hormonal changes.

Mechanisms

Even though there has been research on caloric restriction for over 70 years, the mechanism by which caloric restriction works is still not well understood. Some explanations include reduced core body temperature, reduced cellular divisions, lower metabolic rates, reduced production of free radicals, reduced DNA damage and hormesis.

Temperature

Caloric restriction lowers the core body temperature, a phenomenon believed to be an adaptive response to reduce energy expenditure when nutrients availability is limited. Lowering the temperature may prolong the lifespan of cold blooded animals. Mice, which are warm blooded, have been engineered to have a reduced core body temperature which increased the lifespan independently of calorie restriction.

Hormesis

Some research has pointed toward hormesis as an explanation for the benefits of caloric restriction, representing beneficial actions linked to a low-intensity biological stressor such as reduced calorie intake. As a potential role for caloric restriction, the diet imposes a low-intensity biological stress on the organism, eliciting a defensive response that may help protect it against the disorders of aging. In other words, caloric restriction places the organism in a defensive state so that it can survive adversity, resulting in improved health and longer life. This switch to a defensive state may be controlled by longevity genes.

Mitochondrial Hormesis

Mitochondrial hormesis was a purely hypothetical concept until late 2007, when work on a small worm named Caenorhabditis elegans suggested that the restriction of glucose metabolism extends life span primarily by increasing oxidative stress to stimulate the organism into having an ultimately increased resistance to further oxidative stress. This is probably the first experimental evidence for hormesis being the reason for extended life span following caloric restriction.

Although aging can be conceptualized as the accumulation of damage, the more recent determination that free radicals participate in intracellular signaling has made the categorical equation of their effects with "damage" more problematic than was commonly appreciated in the past. It was previously proposed on a hypothetical basis that free radicals may induce an endogenous response culminating in more effective adaptations that protect against exogenous radicals (and possibly other toxic compounds). Sublethal mitochondrial stress with an attendant augmentation of reactive oxygen species may precipitate many of the beneficial alterations in cellular physiology produced by caloric restriction.

Evolution

It has been recently argued that during years of famine, it may be evolutionarily desirable for an organism to avoid reproduction and to up-regulate protective and repair enzyme mechanisms to ensure that it is fit for reproduction in future years. This argument seems to be supported by recent work studying hormones. Prolonged severe CR lowers total serum and free testosterone while increasing sex hormone binding globulin concentrations in humans; these effects are independent of adiposity.

Lowering of the concentration of insulin and substances related to insulin, such as insulin-like growth factor 1 and growth hormone, has been shown to up-regulate autophagy, the repair mechanism of the cell. A related hypothesis suggests that caloric restriction works by decreasing insulin levels and thereby up-regulating autophagy, but caloric restriction affects many other health indicators, and it is still undecided whether insulin is the main concern. Calorie restriction has been shown to increase DHEA in primates, but it has not been shown to increase DHEA in post-pubescent primates. The extent to which these findings apply to humans is still under investigation.

Chromatin and PHA-4

Evidence suggests that the biological effects of caloric restriction are closely related to chromatin function. One study determined that the gene PHA-4 is responsible for the longevity behind calorie restriction in roundworms, "with similar results expected in humans".

Reduced DNA Damage

Sohal et al. observed that caloric restriction decreased 8-OHdG damages in the DNA of mice heart, skeletal muscle, brain, liver and kidney. The levels of 8-OHdG in the DNA of these organs in 15 month old mice were reduced to an average of 81% of that in the DNA of mice fed an unrestricted diet. Kaneko et al. observed that, in rats, dietary restriction retarded the onset of age-related increases in 8-OHdG in nuclear DNA of brain, heart, liver and kidney. The level of 8-OHdG in these organs of the calorie restricted rats at 30 months averaged 65% of the level in rats fed an unrestricted diet.

In rodents, calorie restriction slows aging, decreases ROS production and reduces the accumulation of oxidative DNA damage in multiple organs. These results link reduced oxidative DNA damage to slower aging. The consistent observation that calorie restriction reduces oxidative DNA damage lends support to the possibility that oxidative DNA damage is associated with aging.

Sirtuin-mediated Mechanism

Sirtuins, specifically Sir2 (found in yeast) has been implicated in the aging of yeast and is a highly conserved, NAD^+ - dependent histone deacetylase. Sir2 homologs have been identified in a wide range of organisms from bacteria to humans. Yeast has 3 SIR genes (SIR2, SIR3, and SIR4) that are responsible for silencing mating type loci, telomeres, and rDNA. Although all three genes are required for the silencing of mating type loci and telomeres, only SIR2 has been implicated in the silencing of rDNA. In addition, SIR2 related genes also regulate formation of some specialized survival forms, such as spores in yeast and daher larvae in *C. elegans*. A study done by Kaeberlein et al. (1999) in yeast found that deletions of Sir2 decreased lifespan, and additional copies increased lifespan.

In many calorie restriction studies, it is believed that Sir2 mediates the longevity effects from calorie restriction for several reasons. First, it was found that in yeast without SIR2, calorie restriction did not impart longevity in yeast; second, in Sir2 mutants an abundance of extra-chromosomal ribosomal DNA circles (that typically limit lifespan) has been observed, and that mitigation of these circles restore regular life span, but still are resistant to calorie restriction-mediated longevity; third, that caloric restriction increases the activity of Sir2 *in vivo*. Although Sir2 has been implicated in calorie restriction-mediated longevity, the method by which Sir2 is regulated under caloric restriction is still debated.

Two hypotheses of Sir2/caloric restriction -mediated longevity is the NADH mechanism and the NAD salvage pathway mechanism. In the NADH hypothesis, it is believed that caloric restriction causes an increase in respiration, which in turn causes a reduction in the levels of NADH. This decrease in the concentration of NADH would up regulate SIR2, since NADH functions as a competitive inhibitor of SIR2. In addition, it has been shown that overexpression of NADH hydrogenase increased longevity and knocking out the electron transport chain blocked caloric restriction-mediated longevity. The NAD salvage pathway mechanism relies on a study by Anderson et al., in which they showed that caloric restriction causes an up regulation of PNC1 (an enzyme responsible for synthesizing NAD from nicotinamide and ADP-ribose) decreases the levels of nicotinamide, which in turn upregulates SIR2 and thus increases lifespan. Although these models are not mutually exclusive, no experiment has been conducted linking the two.

Caloric Restriction Mimetics

Work on the mechanisms of caloric restriction has given hope to the synthesizing of future drugs to increase the human lifespan by simulating the effects of calorie restriction. In particular, the large number of genes and pathways reported to regulate the actions of caloric restriction in model organisms represent attractive targets for developing drugs that mimic the benefits of CR without its side effects.

Sir2, or "silent information regulator 2", is a sirtuin, discovered in baker's yeast cells, that is hypothesized to suppress DNA instability. In mammals, Sir2 is known as SIRT1. One proponent of the view that the gene Sir2 may underlie the effect of calorie restriction in mammals by protecting cells from dying under stress. It is suggested that a low-calorie diet that requires less Nicotinamide adenine dinucleotide to metabolize may allow SIRT1 to be more active in its life-extending processes, possibly by a mechanism of SIRT1 releasing fat from storage cells.

Sirtuins

Attempts are being made to develop drugs that act as CR mimetics, and much of that work has focused on a class of proteins called sirtuins. Resveratrol has been reported to activate SIRT1 and extend the lifespan of yeast, nematode worms, fruit flies, vertebrate fish, and mice consuming a high-caloric diet. However, resveratrol does not extend life span in normal mice and the effect of resveratrol on lifespan in nematodes and fruit flies has been disputed.

There are studies that indicate that resveratrol may not function through SIRT1 but may work through other targets. A clinical trial of the resveratrol formulation SRT501 was suspended.

History

The first person to promote calorie restriction as a means of prolonging life was Luigi Cornaro, a 15th-century Venetian nobleman who adopted a calorie restricted diet at age 35 to address his failing health. It is said his restricted diet cured him of all of his ailments in less than a year, and he went on to live to be 102 years old. His book *Discorsi della vita sobria* (Discourses On the Temperate Life) described his regimen, which centered on the "quantifying principle" of restricting himself to only 350 grams of food daily (including bread, egg yolk, meat, and soup) and 414 milliliters of wine. The book was extremely successful, and "was a true reconceptualization of old age. As late as the Renaissance it was largely the negative aspects of this phase of life which were emphasized... Cornaro's method offered the possibility for the first time not only of a long but also a worthwhile life."

The findings have since been accepted and generalized to a range of other animals. Researchers are investigating the possibility of parallel physiological links in non-human primates and humans. In response to these results, a small number of people have independently adopted the practice of calorie restriction in some form as a potential anti-aging intervention.

Through 2017, the US National Institute on Aging is conducting human clinical trials on caloric restriction to determine potential for reducing the risks of age-related disorders.

Research

Primates

In a 2017 collaborative report on rhesus monkeys by scientists of the US National Institute on Aging and the University of Wisconsin, caloric restriction in the presence of adequate nutrition was effective in delaying the effects of aging. Older age of onset, female gender, lower body weight and fat mass, reduced food intake, diet quality, and lower fasting blood glucose levels were factors associated with fewer disorders of aging and with improved survival rates. Specifically, reduced food intake was beneficial in adult and older primates, but not in younger monkeys. The study indicated that caloric restriction provided health benefits with fewer age-related disorders in elderly monkeys and, because rhesus monkeys are genetically similar to humans, the benefits and mechanisms of caloric restriction may apply to human health during aging.

Rodents

It has been known since the 1930s that reducing the number of calories fed to laboratory rodents increases their life spans. The life extension varies for each species, but on average there was a 30–40% increase in life span in both mice and rats. In late adulthood, acute CR partially or completely reverses age-related alterations of liver, brain and heart proteins, and mice placed on CR at 19 months of age show an increases in life span.

Yeast

Fungi models are very easy to manipulate, and many crucial steps toward the understanding of aging have been made with them. Many studies were undertaken on budding yeast and fission yeast to analyze the cellular mechanisms behind increased longevity due to calorie restriction. First, calorie restriction is often called dietary restriction because the same effects on life span can be achieved by only changing the nutrient quality without changing the number of calories. Data from Guarente and others showed that genetic manipulations in nutrient-signaling pathways could mimic the effects of dietary restriction. In some cases, dietary restriction requires mitochondrial respiration to increase longevity (chronological aging), and in some other cases not (replicative aging). Nutrient sensing in yeast controls stress defense, mitochondrial functions, Sir2, and others. These functions are all known to regulate aging. Genes involved in these mechanisms are TOR, PKA, SCH9, MSN2/4, RIM15, and SIR2. Importantly, yeast responses to CR can be modulated by genetic background. Therefore, while some strains respond to calorie restriction with increased lifespan, in others calorie restriction shortens it

Humans

Studies have been conducted to examine the effects of calorie restriction with adequate intake of nutrients in humans; however, long-term effects are unknown.

Biomarkers for Cardiovascular Risk

A review of the effects of calorie restriction on the aging heart and vasculature concluded that "Data from animal and human studies indicate that [beyond the effects of "implementation of healthier diets and regular exercise"], more drastic interventions, i.e., calorie restriction with adequate nutrition (CRAN), may have additional beneficial effects on several metabolic and molecular factors that are modulating cardiovascular aging itself (e.g., cardiac and arterial stiffness and heart rate variability)." Studies of long-term practitioners of rigorous calorie restriction show that their risk factors for atherosclerosis are substantially improved in a manner consistent with experimental studies in rodent models of atherosclerosis and nonhuman primates. Risk factors such as c-reactive protein; serum triglycerides, low-density lipoprotein, high-density lipoprotein; blood pressure; and fasting blood sugar, are substantially more favorable than persons consuming usual Western diets and comparable or better than long-term endurance exercisers. Similar effects were also seen during a "natural experiment" in Biosphere 2, and in subjects in the "Minnesota Starvation Experiment" during World War II. Cardiac "diastolic function was better in subjects who practiced strict calorie restriction for 3–15 years than that in healthy age- and sex-matched control subjects ... calorie restriction subjects had less ventricular stiffness and less viscous loss of diastolic recoil, both of which would be consistent with less myocardial fibrosis. "These effects, in combination with other benefits of calorie restriction, such as protection against obesity, diabetes, hypertension, and cancer, suggest that CR may have a major beneficial effect on health span, life span, and quality of life in humans."

Biomarkers for Cancer Risk

Long-term calorie restriction in humans results in a reduction of several metabolic and hormonal factors that have been associated with increased risk of some of the most common types of cancer in developed countries, consistent with similar shifts in calorie restriction rodents and nonhuman primates, in whom calorie restriction affords substantial protection against cancer morbidity and mortality. These include lower levels of total and abdominal fat, circulating insulin, testosterone, estradiol, and inflammatory cytokines linked to cancer. Long-term calorie restriction can also reduce levels of serum Insulin-like growth factor 1 in humans, and increase levels of IGFBP-3; however, unlike in rodents, this effect can be blocked if dietary protein is not reduced to the Dietary Reference Intake.

Concerns and Confounders

Activity Levels

Calorie restriction preserves muscle tissue in nonhuman primates and rodents. Mechanisms include reduced muscle cell apoptosis and inflammation; protection against or adaptation to age-related mitochondrial abnormalities; and preserved muscle stem cell function. Muscle tissue grows when stimulated, so it has been suggested that the calorie-restricted test animals exercised more than their companions on higher calories, perhaps because animals enter a foraging state during calorie restriction. However, studies show that overall activity levels are no higher in calorie restriction than ad libitum animals in youth, while calorie restriction animals are more active at middle age and beyond due to a protective effect against the decline in activity observed in middle-aged and older animals.

Laboratory rodents placed on a calorie restriction diet tend to exhibit increased activity levels (particularly when provided with exercise equipment) at feeding time. Monkeys undergoing calorie restriction also appear more restless immediately before and after meals. Despite this brief daily period of increased activity overall activity is no higher in calorie restriction than ad libitum animals in youth after an initial period of adaptation to the diet. On the other hand, calorie restriction has been found to retard the *decline* in activity that occurs during normal aging: in one study, animals on a conventional diet "showed little activity" by early middle age, while those on calorie restriction "were observed to run around the cage and climb onto and hang from the wire cage tops throughout their life spans. In fact, the longest surviving calorie restriction mouse was observed hanging from the top of his cage only 3 days before he became moribund."

Larger Organisms

Another objection to calorie restriction as an advisable lifestyle for humans is the claim that the physiological mechanisms that determine longevity are very complex, and that the effect would be small to negligible in our species. Several of the biological changes observed in animals with longer life spans on calorie restriction have already been observed in humans which proponents argue suggests that the life-extending properties of calorie restriction will extend to humans.

Stereotyped Behavior

Observations in some accounts of animals undergoing calorie restriction have noted an increase in stereotyped behaviors. For example, monkeys on calorie restriction have demonstrated an increase in licking, sucking, and rocking behavior.

Aggression

A calorie restriction regimen may also lead to increased aggressive behavior in animals.

Obese Controls

It has sometimes been suggested that the lives of calorie-restricted animals are only extended relative to control animals whose lives are artificially shortened by weight-gain from unnatural ad libitum feeding in the laboratory. However, studies designed to test this hypothesis suggest that reduced fat mass is not a major contributor to the longevity effects of calorie restriction. The strongest evidence comes from a study in which ob/ob mice, which are genetically prone to overeating and obesity, were compared to lean mice of the same genetic background but lacking the ob/ob mutation. When placed on calorie restriction, the ob/ob mice still have over twice the fat mass of ad libitum-fed congenic lean mice, and yet they have double the lifespan. Additionally, many modern calorie restriction studies restrict the control animals by 10–20% below their ad libitum intake in order to avoid confounding by obesity.

Overweight

Overweight is having more body fat than is optimally healthy. Being overweight is common especially where food supplies are plentiful and lifestyles are sedentary.

Excess weight has reached epidemic proportions globally, with more than 1 billion adults being either overweight or obese in 2003. In 2013 this increased to more than 2 billion. Increases have been observed across all age groups.

A healthy body requires a minimum amount of fat for proper functioning of the hormonal, reproductive, and immune systems, as thermal insulation, as shock absorption for sensitive areas, and as energy for future use. But the accumulation of too much storage fat can impair movement, flexibility, and alter appearance of the body.

Classification

The degree to which a person is overweight is generally described by body mass index (BMI). Overweight is defined as a BMI of 25 or more, thus it includes pre-obesity defined as a BMI between 25 and 30 and obesity as defined by a BMI of 30 or more. Pre obese and overweight however are often used interchangeably thus giving overweight a common definition of a BMI of between 25 -30. There are however several other common ways to measure the amount of adiposity or fat present in an individual's body.

- Body mass index

  The body mass index (BMI) is a measure of a person's weight taking into account their height. It is given by the formula: BMI equals a person's weight (mass) in kilograms divided by the square of the person's height in metres. The units therefore are kg/m^2 but BMI measures are typically used and written without units.

  BMI provides a significantly more accurate representation of body fat content than simply measuring a person's weight. It is only moderately correlated with both body fat percentage and body fat mass (R^2 of 0.68). It does not take into account certain factors such as pregnancy or bodybuilding; however, the BMI is an accurate reflection of fat percentage in the majority of the adult population.

- Body volume index

  The body volume index (BVI) was devised in 2000 as a computer, rather than manual, measurement of the human body for obesity and an alternative to the BMI

  Body volume index uses 3D software to create an accurate 3D image of a person so BVI can differentiate between people with the same BMI rating, but who have a different shape and different weight distribution.

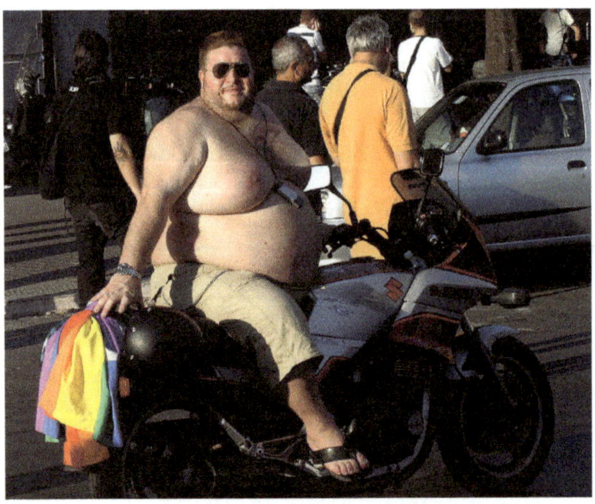

An obese man on a motorcycle

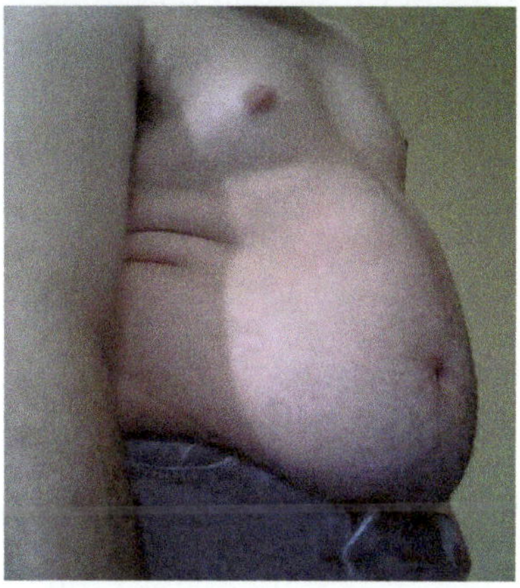

Belly of an overweight teenager.

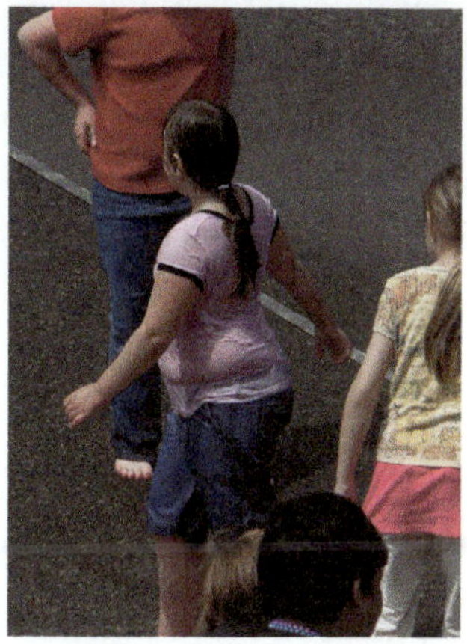

Children with varying levels of body fat

BVI measures where a person's weight and the fat are located on the body, rather than total weight or total fat content and places emphasis on the weight carried around the abdomen, commonly known as central obesity. There has been an acceptance in recent years that abdominal fat and weight around the abdomen constitute a greater health risk.

- Simple weighing

  The person's weight is measured and compared to an estimated ideal weight. This is the easiest and most common method, but by far the least accurate, as it only measures one quantity (weight) and often does not take into account many factors such as height, body type, and relative amount of muscle mass.

- Skinfold calipers or "pinch test"

  The skin at several specific points on the body is pinched and the thickness of the resulting fold is measured. This measures the thickness of the layers of fat located under the skin, from which a general measurement of total amount of fat in the body is calculated. This method can be reasonably accurate for many people, but it assumes particular fat distribution patterns over the body—which may not apply to all individuals, and does not account for fat deposits not directly under the skin. Also, as the measurement and analysis generally involves a high degree of practice and interpretation, an accurate result requires that a professional perform it. It cannot generally be done by patients themselves.

- Bioelectrical impedance analysis

  A small electric current is passed through the body to measure its electrical resistance. As fat and muscle conduct electricity differently, this method can provide a direct measurement of the body fat percentage, in relation to muscle mass. In the past, this technique could only be performed reliably by trained professionals with specialized equipment, but it is now possible to buy home testing kits that let people do this themselves with a minimum of training. Despite the improved simplicity of this process over the years, however, a number of factors can affect the results, including hydration and body temperature, so it still needs some care when taking the test to ensure that the results are accurate.

- Hydrostatic weighing

  Considered one of the more accurate methods of measuring body fat, this technique involves complete submersion of a person in water, with special equipment to measure the person's weight while submerged. This weight is then compared with "dry weight" as recorded outside the water to determine overall body density. As fat is less dense than muscle, careful application of this technique can provide a reasonably close estimate of fat content in the body. This technique does, however, require expensive specialized equipment and trained professionals to administer it properly.

- Dual-energy X-ray absorptiometry (DEXA)

  Originally developed to measure bone density, DEXA imaging is also used to precisely determine body fat content by using the density of various body tissues to identify which portions of the body are fat. This test is generally considered very accurate, but requires a great deal of expensive medical equipment and trained professionals to perform.

The most common method for discussing this subject and the one used primarily by researchers and advisory institutions is BMI. Definitions of what is considered overweight vary by ethnicity. The current definition proposed by the US National Institutes of Health (NIH) and the World Health Organization (WHO) designates whites, Hispanics and blacks with a BMI of 25 or more as overweight. For Asians, overweight is a BMI between 23 and 29.9 and obesity for all groups is a BMI of 30 or more.

BMI, however, does not account extremes of muscle mass, some rare genetic factors, the very young, and a few other individual variations. Thus it is possible for an individuals with a BMI of less than 25 to have excess body fat, while others may have a BMI that is significantly higher without falling into this category. Some of the above methods for determining body fat are more accurate than BMI but come with added complexity.

If an individual is overweight and has excess body fat it could, but will not always, create or lead to health risks. Reports are surfacing, however, that being mildly overweight to slightly obese – BMI being between 24 and 31.9 – may be actually beneficial and that people with BMI between 24 and 31.9 could actually live longer than normal weight or underweight persons.

Health Effects

While the negative health outcomes associated with obesity are accepted within the medical community, the health implications of the overweight category are more controversial. The generally accepted view is that being overweight causes similar health problems to obesity, but to a lesser degree. A 2016 review estimated that the risk of death increases by 7 percent among overweight people with a BMI of 25 to 27.5 and 20 percent among overweight people with a BMI of 27.5 to 30. The Framingham heart study found that being overweight at age 40 reduced life expectancy by three years. Being overweight also increases the risk of oligospermia and azoospermia in men.

Katherine Flegal et al., however, found that the mortality rate for individuals who are classified as overweight (BMI 25 to 30) may actually be lower than for those with an "ideal" weight (BMI 18.5 to 25).

Being overweight has been identified as a cause of cancer, and is projected to overtake smoking as the primary cause of cancer in developed countries as cases of cancer linked to smoking dwindle.

Psychological well-being is also at risk in the overweight individual due to social discrimination. However, children under the age of eight are normally not affected.

Being overweight has been shown not to increase mortality in older people: in a study of 70 to 75-year old Australians, mortality was lowest for "overweight" individuals (BMI 25 to 30), while a study of Koreans found that, among those initially aged 65 or more, an increase in BMI to above 25 was not associated with increased risk of death.

Causes

Being overweight is generally caused by the intake of more calories (by eating) than are expended by the body (by exercise and everyday living). Factors that may contribute to this imbalance include:

- Alcoholism
- Eating disorders (such as binge eating)
- Genetic predisposition
- Hormonal imbalances (e.g. hypothyroidism)
- Insufficient or poor-quality sleep
- Limited physical exercise and sedentary lifestyle
- Poor nutrition

- Metabolic disorders, which could be caused by repeated attempts to lose weight by weight cycling
- Overeating
- Psychotropic medication (e.g. olanzapine)
- Smoking cessation and other stimulant withdrawal
- Stress

People who have insulin dependant diabetes and chronically overdose insulin may gain weight, while people who already are overweight may develop insulin tolerance, and in the long run type II diabetes.

Treatment

The usual treatments for overweight individuals is diet and physical exercise.

Dietitians generally recommend eating several balanced meals dispersed through the day, with a combination of progressive, primarily aerobic, physical exercise.

Because these general treatments help most case of obesity, they are common in all levels of overweight individuals.

Epidemiology

As much as 64% of the United States adult population is considered either overweight or obese, and this percentage has increased over the last four decades.

Hypervitaminosis

Hypervitaminosis refers to a condition of abnormally high storage levels of vitamins, which can lead to toxic symptoms. The medical names of the different conditions are derived from the vitamin involved: an excess of vitamin A, for example, is called hypervitaminosis A.

Hypervitaminosis primarily affects the fat soluble vitamins, as these are stored by the body for longer period than the water-soluble vitamins. However, avoiding excesses of both classes of vitamins can make the condition hard to get.

Generally, toxic levels of vitamins stem from high supplement intake and not from natural food. Toxicities of fat-soluble vitamins can also be caused by a large intake of highly fortified foods, but natural food rarely deliver dangerous levels of fat-soluble vitamins. Liver is a natural food which can cause toxic levels of vitamin A; vegetable sources of vitamin A will not cause toxic levels of vitamin A.

The Dietary Reference Intake recommendations from the United States Department of Agriculture define a "tolerable upper intake level" for most vitamins.

High dosage vitamin A; high dosage, slow release vitamin B_3; and very high dosage vitamin B_6 alone (i.e. without vitamin B complex) are sometimes associated with vitamin side effects that usually rapidly cease with supplement reduction or cessation.

Fat Soluble

With few exceptions, like some vitamins from B complex, hypervitaminosis usually occurs more with fat-soluble vitamins (D, E, K and A or 'DEKA'), which are stored in the liver and fatty tissues of the body. These vitamins build up and remain for a longer time in the body than water-soluble vitamins.

Conditions include:

- Hypervitaminosis A
- Hypervitaminosis D
- Hypervitaminosis E
- Hypervitaminosis K, unique as the true upper limit is less clear as is its bioavailability.

According to Williams' Essentials of Diet and Nutrition Therapy it is difficult to set a DRI for vitamin K because part of the requirement can be met by intestinal bacterial synthesis.

- Reliable information is lacking as to the vitamin K content of many foods or its bioavailability. With this in mind the Expert Committee established an AI rather than an RDA.
- This RDA (AI for men age 19 and older is 120 µg/day, AI for women is 90 µg/day) is adequate to preserve blood clotting, but the correct intake needed for optimum bone health is unknown. Toxicity has not been reported.

Minerals

High doses of mineral supplements can also lead to side effects and toxicity. Mineral-supplement poisoning does occur occasionally, most often due to excessive intake of iron-containing supplements.

Comparative Safety Statistics

In the United States, overdose exposure to all formulations of "vitamins" was reported by 62,562 individuals in 2004 (nearly 80% [~78%, n=48,989] of these exposures were in children under the age of 6), leading to 53 "major" life-threatening outcomes and 3 deaths (2 from vitamins D and E; 1 from polyvitaminic type formula, with iron and no fluoride). This may be compared to the 19,250 people who died of unintentional poisoning of all kinds in the U.S. in the same year (2004). In 2010, 71,000 exposures to various vitamins and multivitamin-mineral formulations were reported to poison control centers, which resulted in 15 major reactions but no deaths.

Before 1998, several deaths per year were associated with pharmaceutical iron-containing supplements, especially brightly colored, sugar-coated, high-potency iron supplements, and most deaths were children. Unit packaging restrictions on supplements with more than 30 mg of iron have since reduced deaths to 0 or 1 per year. These statistics compare with 59 confirmed deaths due to aspirin poisoning in 2003 and 147 deaths known to be associated with acetaminophen-containing products in 2003.

Hypervitaminosis A

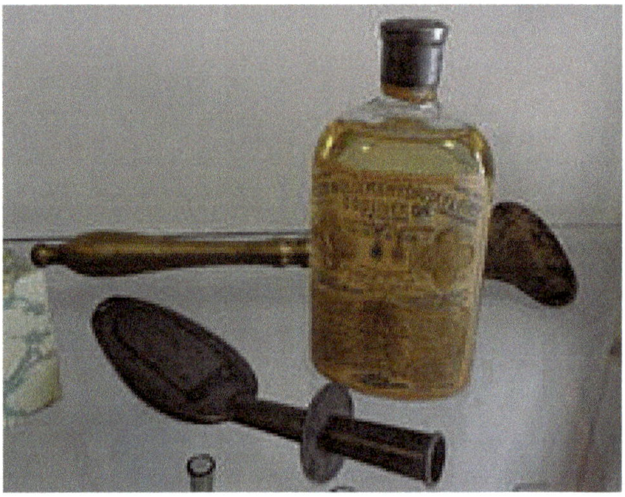

Cod liver oil - a potentially toxic source of Vitamin A: Hypervitaminosis A can result from ingestion of too much vitamin A from diet, supplements, or prescription medications.

Hypervitaminosis A refers to the toxic effects of ingesting too much preformed vitamin A. Symptoms arise as a result of altered bone metabolism and altered metabolism of other fat-soluble vitamins. Hypervitaminosis A is believed to have occurred in early humans, and the problem has persisted throughout human history.

Toxicity results from ingesting too much preformed vitamin A from foods (such as fish or animal liver), supplements, or prescription medications and can be prevented by ingesting no more than the recommended daily amount.

Diagnosis can be difficult, as serum retinol is not sensitive to toxic levels of vitamin A, but there are effective tests available. Hypervitaminosis A is usually treated by stopping intake of the offending food(s), supplement(s), or medication. Most people make a full recovery.

High intake of provitamin carotenoids (such as beta carotene) from vegetables and fruits does not cause hypervitaminosis A, as conversion from carotenoids to the active form of vitamin A is regulated by the body to maintain an optimum level of the vitamin. Carotenoids themselves cannot produce toxicity.

Signs and Symptoms

Symptoms may include:

- Abnormal softening of the skull bone (craniotabes—infants and children)
- Blurred vision
- Bone pain or swelling
- Bulging fontanelle (infants)
- Changes in consciousness
- Decreased appetite
- Dizziness
- Double vision (young children)
- Drowsiness
- Headache
- Gastric mucosal calcinosis
- Heart valve calcification
- Hypercalcemia
- Increased intracranial pressure manifesting as cerebral edema, papilledema, and headache (may be referred to as Idiopathic intracranial hypertension)
- Irritability
- Liver damage
- Nausea
- Poor weight gain (infants and children)
- Skin and hair changes
- Cracking at corners of the mouth

- Hair loss
- Higher sensitivity to sunlight
- Oily skin and hair (seborrhea)
- Premature epiphyseal closure
- Skin peeling, itching
- Spontaneous fracture
- Yellow discoloration of the skin (aurantiasis cutis)
- Uremic pruritus
- Vision changes
- Vomiting

Causes

Hypervitaminosis A results from excessive intake of preformed vitamin A. A genetic variance in tolerance to vitamin A intake may occur. Children are particularly sensitive to vitamin A, with daily intakes of 1500 IU/kg body weight reportedly leading to toxicity.

Types of Vitamin A

- Provitamin carotenoids - such as beta carotene - are "largely impossible" to cause toxicity, as their conversion to retinol is highly regulated. No vitamin A toxicity has ever been reported from ingestion of excessive amounts. Overconsumption of beta carotene can only cause carotenosis, a harmless and reversible cosmetic condition in which the skin turns orange.
- Preformed vitamin A absorption and storage in the liver occur very efficiently until a pathologic condition develops. When ingested, 70-90% of preformed vitamin A is absorbed and used.

Sources of Toxicity

- Diet - liver is high in vitamin A. The liver of certain animals — including the polar bear, bearded seal, walrus, moose, — are particularly toxic.
- Supplements - usually when taken above recommended dosages - can be toxic. Cod liver oil is particularly high in vitamin A.
- Medications - at high doses of vitamin A - are often used on long-term basis in

numerous preventive and therapeutic medical applications, which may lead to hypervitaminosis A.

Types of Toxicity

- Acute toxicity occurs over a period of hours or a few days, and is less of a problem than chronic toxicity.
- Chronic toxicity - ingestion of high amounts of preformed vitamin A for months or years - results from daily intakes greater than 25,000 IU for 6 years or longer and more than 100,000 IU for 6 months or longer - are considered toxic.

Mechanism

Absorption and storage in the liver of preformed vitamin A occur very efficiently until a pathologic condition develops.

Delivery to Tissues

Absorption

When ingested, 70-90% of preformed vitamin A is absorbed and used.

Storage

80-90% of the total body reserves of vitamin A are in the liver (with 80-90% of this amount being stored in hepatic stellate cells and the remaining 10-20% being stored in hepatocytes). Fat is another significant storage site, while the lung and kidneys may also be capable of storage.

Transport

Until recently, it was thought that the sole important retinoid delivery pathway to tissues involved retinol bound to retinol-binding protein (RBP4). More recent findings, however, indicate that retinoids can be delivered to tissues through multiple overlapping delivery pathways, involving chylomicrons, very low density lipoprotein (VLDL) and low density lipoprotein (LDL), retinoic acid bound to albumin, water soluble β-glucuronides of retinol and retinoic acid, and provitamin A carotenoids.

The range of serum retinol concentrations under normal conditions is 1–3 μmol/l. Elevated amounts of retinyl ester (i.e., > 10% of total circulating vitamin A) in the fasting state have been used as markers for chronic hypervitaminosis A in humans. Candidate mechanisms for this increase include decreased hepatic uptake of vitamin A and the leaking of esters into the bloodstream from saturated hepatic stellate cells.

Effects

Effects include increased bone turnover and altered metabolism of fat-soluble vitamins. More research is needed to fully elucidate the effects.

Increased Bone Turnover

Retinoic acid suppresses osteoblast activity and stimulates osteoclast formation *in vitro*, resulting in increased bone resorption and decreased bone formation. It is likely to exert this effect by binding to specific nuclear receptors (members of the retinoic acid receptor or retinoid X receptor nuclear transcription family) which are found in every cell (including osteoblasts and osteoclasts).

This change in bone turnover is likely to be the reason for numerous effects seen in hypervitaminosis A, such as hypercalcemia and numerous bone changes such as bone loss that potentially leads to osteoporosis, spontaneous bone fractures, altered skeletal development in children, skeletal pain, radiographic changes, and bone lesions.

Altered Fat-soluble Vitamin Metabolism

Vitamin A is fat-soluble and high levels have been reported affect metabolism of the other fat-soluble vitamins D, E, and K.

The toxic effects of vitamin A might be related to altered vitamin D metabolism, concurrent ingestion of substantial amounts of vitamin D, or binding of vitamin A to receptor heterodimers. Antagonistic and synergistic interactions between these two vitamins have been reported, as they relate to skeletal health.

Stimulation of bone resorption by vitamin A has been reported to be independent of its effects on vitamin D.

Mitochondrial Toxicity

Vitamin A exerts several toxic effects regarding redox environment and mitochondrial function

Diagnosis

Tests

Tests may include:

- bone X-rays
- blood calcium test
- cholesterol test

- liver function test
- blood test for vitamin A

Relevance of Blood Tests

Retinol Concentrations are Nonsensitive Indicators

Assessing vitamin A status in persons with subtoxicity or toxicity is complicated because serum retinol concentrations are not sensitive indicators in this range of liver vitamin A reserves. The range of serum retinol concentrations under normal conditions is 1–3 μmol/l and, because of homeostatic regulation, that range varies little with widely disparate vitamin A intakes

Retinol Esters Have Been used as Markers

Retinyl esters can be distinguished from retinol in serum and other tissues and quantified with the use of methods such as high-performance liquid chromatography.

Elevated amounts of retinyl ester (i.e., > 10% of total circulating vitamin A) in the fasting state have been used as markers for chronic hypervitaminosis A in humans and monkeys. This increased retinyl ester may be due to decreased hepatic uptake of vitamin A and the leaking of esters into the bloodstream from saturated hepatic stellate cells.

Prevention

Hypervitaminosis A can be prevented by not ingesting more than the US Institute of Medicine Daily Tolerable Upper Level of intake for Vitamin A. This level is for synthetic and natural retinol ester forms of vitamin A. Carotene forms from dietary sources are not toxic. The dose over and above the RDA is among the narrowest of the vitamins and minerals. Possible pregnancy, liver disease, high alcohol consumption, and smoking are indications for close monitoring and limitation of vitamin A administration.

Daily Tolerable Upper Level

Life stage group category	Upper Level (μg/day)
Infants	
0–6 months	600
7–12 months	600
Children	
1–3 years	600
4–8 years	900

Males 9–13 years 14–18 years 19 – >70 years	1700 2800 3000
Females 9–13 years 14–18 years 19 – >70 years	1700 2800 3000
Pregnancy <19 years 19 – >50 years	2800 3000
Lactation <19 years 19 – >50 years	2800 3000

Treatment

- Stopping high Vitamin A intake is the standard treatment. Most people fully recover.
- Phosphatidylcholine (in the form of PPC or DLPC), the substrate for Lecithin retinol acyltransferase, which converts retinol into Retinyl esters (the storage forms of vitamin A).
- Vitamin E may alleviate hypervitaminosis A.
- Liver transplantation may be a valid option if no improvement occurs.

If liver damage has progressed into fibrosis, synthesizing capacity is compromised and supplementation can replenish PC. However, recovery is dependent on removing the causative agent; stopping high Vitamin A intake.

History

Vitamin A toxicity is known to be an ancient phenomenon; fossilized skeletal remains of early humans suggest bone abnormalities may have been caused by hypervitaminosis A.

Vitamin A toxicity has long been known to the Inuit and has been known by Europeans since at least 1597 when Gerrit de Veer wrote in his diary that, while taking refuge in the winter in Nova Zemlya, he and his men became severely ill after eating polar bear liver.

In 1913, Antarctic explorers Douglas Mawson and Xavier Mertz were both poisoned (and Mertz died) from eating the livers of their sled dogs during the Far Eastern Party. Another study suggests, however, that exhaustion and diet change are more likely to have caused the tragedy.

Other Animals

Some Arctic animals demonstrate no signs of hypervitaminosis A despite having 10-20 times the level of vitamin A in their livers as other Arctic animals. These animals are top predators and include the polar bear, Arctic fox, bearded seal, and glaucous gull. This ability to efficiently store higher amounts of vitamin A may have contributed to their survival in the extreme environment of the Arctic.

Hypervitaminosis A causes hypothyroidism in mouse.

Treatment

These treatments have been used to help treat or manage toxicity in animals. Although not considered part of standard treatment, they might be of some benefit to humans.

- Vitamin E appears to be an effective treatment in rabbits, prevents side effects in chicks
- Taurine significantly reduces toxic effects in rats. Retinoids can be conjugated by taurine and other substances. Significant amounts of retinotaurine are excreted in the bile, and this retinol conjugate is thought to be an excretory form, as it has little biological activity.
- Cholestin - significantly reduces toxic effects in rats.
- Vitamin K prevents hypoprothrombinemia in rats and can sometimes control the increase in plasma/cell ratios of vitamin A.

Hypervitaminosis D

Hypervitaminosis D is a state of vitamin D toxicity. The normal range for blood concentration is 30.0 to 74.0 nanograms per milliliter (ng/mL).

Signs and Symptoms

An excess of vitamin D causes abnormally high blood concentrations of calcium, which can cause overcalcification of the bones, soft tissues, heart and kidneys. In addition, hypertension can result. Symptoms of vitamin D toxicity may include the following:

- Dehydration
- Vomiting
- Decreased appetite
- Irritability
- Constipation
- Fatigue
- Muscle weakness
- Metastatic calcification of the soft tissues

Hypervitaminosis D symptoms appear several months after excessive doses of vitamin D are administered. In almost every case, a low-calcium diet combined with corticosteroid drugs will allow for a full recovery within a month. There is a theory that some of the symptoms of vitamin D toxicity are actually due to vitamin K depletion. One animal experiment has demonstrated that co-consumption with vitamin K reduced adverse effects. Has not been tested in humans.

Recommended Supplement Limits

The U.S Institute of Medicine has established a Tolerable Upper Intake Level (UL) to protect against vitamin D toxicity. These levels in microgram (mcg or µg) and International Units (IU) for male and female are:

(Conversion : 1 µg = 40 IU and 0.025 µg = 1 IU.)

- 0–6 months: 25 µg (1000 IU)
- 7–12 months: 38 µg (1500 IU)
- 1–3 years: 63 µg (2500 IU)
- 4–8 years:75 µg (3000 IU)
- 9+ years:100 µg (4000 IU)
- Pregnant and Lactating: 100 µg (4000 IU)

The recommended dietary allowance is 15 µg/d (600 IU per day; 800 IU for those over 70 years). Overdose has been observed at 1,925 µg/d (77,000 IU per day). Acute overdose requires between 15,000 µg/d (600,000 IU per day) and 42,000 µg/d (1,680,000 IU per day) over a period of several days to months.

Suggested Tolerable Upper Intake Level (UL)

Based on risk assessment, a safe upper intake level of 250 µg (10,000 IU) per day in healthy adult has been suggested by non-government authors. However, no government has a UL higher than 4,000 IU.

Long-term Effects of Supplementary Oral Intake

Excessive exposure to sunlight poses no risk in vitamin D toxicity through overproduction of vitamin D precursor, cholecalciferol, regulating vitamin D production. During ultraviolet exposure, the concentration of vitamin D precursors produced in the skin reach an equilibrium, and any further vitamin D that is produced is degraded. This process is less efficient with increased melanin pigmentation in the skin. Endogenous production with full body exposure to sunlight is comparable to taking an oral dose between 250 μg and 625 μg (10,000 IU and 25,000 IU) per day.

Vitamin D oral supplementation and skin synthesis have a different effect on the transport form of vitamin D, plasma calcifediol concentrations. Endogenously synthesized vitamin D_3 travels mainly with vitamin D-binding protein, which slows hepatic delivery of vitamin D and the availability in the plasma. In contrast, orally administered vitamin D produces rapid hepatic delivery of vitamin D and increases plasma calcifediol.

It has been questioned whether to ascribe a state of sub-optimal vitamin D status when the annual variation in ultraviolet will naturally produce a period of falling levels, and such a seasonal decline has been a part of Europeans' adaptive environment for 1000 generations. Still more contentious is recommending supplementation when those supposedly in need of it arc labeled healthy and serious doubts exist as to the long-term effect of attaining and maintaining serum 25(OH)D of at least 80nmol/L by supplementation.

Current theories of the mechanism behind vitamin D toxicity propose that:

- Intake of vitamin D raises calcitriol concentrations in the plasma and cell
- Intake of vitamin D raises plasma calcifediol concentrations which exceed the binding capacity of the DBP, and free calcifediol enters the cell
- Intake of vitamin D raises the concentration of vitamin D metabolites which exceed DBP binding capacity and free calcitriol enters the cell

All of which affect gene transcription and overwhelm the vitamin D signal transduction process, leading to vitamin D toxicity.

Cardiovascular Disease

Evidence suggests that dietary vitamin D may be carried by lipoprotein particles into cells of the artery wall and atherosclerotic plaque, where it may be converted to active form by monocyte-macrophages. This raises questions regarding the effects of vitamin

D intake on atherosclerotic calcification and cardiovascular risk as it may be causing vascular calcification. Calcifediol is implicated in the etiology of atherosclerosis, especially in non-Caucasians.

The levels of the active form of vitamin D, calcitriol, are inversely correlated with coronary calcification. Moreover, the active vitamin D analog, alfacalcidol, seems to protect patients from developing vascular calcification. Serum vitamin D has been found to correlate with calcified atherosclerotic plaque in African Americans as they have higher active serum vitamin D levels compared to Euro-Americans. Higher levels of calcidiol positively correlate with aorta and carotid calcified atherosclerotic plaque in African Americans but not with coronary plaque, whereas individuals of European descent have an opposite, negative association. There are racial differences in the association of coronary calcified plaque in that there is less calcified atherosclerotic plaque in the coronary arteries of African-Americans than in whites.

A case control study on a population in southern India found that more than 50% of patients with ischaemic heart disease had serum levels of vitamin D higher than 222.5 nmol/L, but the study did not evaluate causation.

Among descent groups with heavy sun exposure during their evolution, taking supplemental vitamin D to attain the 25(OH)D level associated with optimal health in studies done with mainly European populations may have deleterious outcomes. Despite abundant sunshine in India, vitamin D status in Indians are low and suggests a public health need to fortify Indian foods with vitamin D. However, the levels found in India are consistent with many other studies of tropical populations which have found that even an extreme amount of sun exposure, does not raise 25(OH)D levels to the levels typically found in Europeans.

Recommendations stemming for a single standard for optimal serum 25(OH)D concentrations ignores the differing genetically mediated determinates of serum 25(OH)D and may result in ethnic minorities in Western countries having the results of studies done with subjects not representative of ethnic diversity applied to them. Vitamin D levels vary for genetically mediated reasons as well as environmental ones.

Ethnic Differences

Possible ethnic differences in physiological pathways for ingested vitamin D, such as the Inuit, may confound across the board recommendations for vitamin D levels. Inuit compensate for lower production of vitamin D by converting more of this vitamin to its most active form.

A Toronto study of young Canadians of diverse ancestry applied a standard of serum 25(OH)D levels that was significantly higher than official recommendations. These levels were described to be 75 nmol/L as "optimal", between 75 nmol/L and 50 nmol/L as "insufficient" and < 50 nmol/L as "deficient". 22% of individuals of European ancestry had 25(OH)D levels less than the 40 nmol/L cutoff, comparable to the values observed in previous studies (40nmol/L is 15 ng/mL). 78% of individuals of East Asian ancestry and 77% of individuals of South Asian ancestry had 25(OH)D concentrations lower than 40 nmol/L. The East Asians in the Toronto sample had low 25(OH)D levels when compared to whites. In a Chinese population at particular risk for esophageal cancer and with the high serum 25(OH)D concentrations have a significantly increased risk of the precursor lesion.

Studies on the South Asians population uniformly point to low 25(OH)D levels, despite abundant sunshine. Rural men around Delhi average 44nmol/L. Healthy Indians seem have low 25(OH)D levels which are not very different from healthy South Asians living in Canada. South Indian patients with ischemic heart disease have serum 25-hydroxyvitamin D_3 levels which are above 222.5 nmol/l and considered extremely high. Measuring melanin content to assess skin pigmentation showed an inverse relationship with serum 25(OH)D. The uniform occurrence of very low serum 25(OH)D in Indians living in India and Chinese in China does not support the hypothesis that the low levels seen in the more pigmented are due to lack of synthesis from the sun at higher latitudes. A study of French Canadians found that a significant minority did not maximize ingested serum 25(OH)D for genetic reasons; vitamin D-binding protein polymorphisms explained as much of the variation in circulating 25(OH)D as did total ingestion of vitamin D.

Premature Aging

Complex regulatory mechanisms control metabolism. Recent epidemiologic evidence suggests that there is a narrow range of vitamin D levels in which vascular function is optimized. Levels above or below this range increased mortality. Animal research suggests that both excess and deficiency of vitamin D appears to cause abnormal functioning and premature aging.

Hypervitaminosis E

Hypervitaminosis E is a state of vitamin E toxicity. Since vitamin E can act as an anticoagulant and may increase the risk of bleeding problems, many agencies have set a tolerable upper intake levels (UL) for vitamin E at 1,000 mg (1,500 IU) per day. This UL was established due to an increased incidence of hemorrhaging with higher doses of supplemental vitamin E. Doses of vitamin E above the UL can also magnify the anti-platelet effects of certain drugs such as anti-coagulant medications and aspirin, which can cause life-threatening symptoms in ill patients. Hypervitaminosis E may also counteract vitamin K, leading to a vitamin K deficiency.

Signs and Symptoms

- Blotchy skin
- Increased bleeding
- Increased blood level of triglycerides
- Decreased production of thyroid hormones
- Decreased activity of vitamin K
- Increased bleeding from aspirin or anti-coagulant medications

References

- "Effects of sex steroid hormones on regional fat depots as assessed by magnetic resonance imaging in transsexuals". Ajpendo.physiology.org. 1999-02-01. Retrieved 2013-01-05
- Gower BA, Casazza K (October–December 2013). "Divergent Effects of Obesity on Bone Health". Journal of Clinical Densitometry. 16 (4): 450–454. PMID 24063845. doi:10.1016/j.jocd.2013.08.010
- Spindler, Stephen R. (2010). "Biological Effects of Calorie Restriction: Implications for Modification of Human Aging". The Future of Aging. pp. 367–438. ISBN 978-90-481-3998-9. doi:10.1007/978-90-481-3999-6_12
- "Iron Toxicity, What You Don't Know". Plants Poisonous to Livestock. Cornell University Department of Animal Science. Retrieved 2012-04-09
- Valentine, Kevin; Mastropietro, Christopher; Sarnaik, Ashok P. "Infantile iron poisoning: Challenges in diagnosis and management". Pediatric Critical Care Medicine. 10 (3): e31–e33. doi:10.1097/pcc.0b013e318198b0c2
- "Researchers weigh risks due to overweight". CA: A Cancer Journal for Clinicians. 55 (5): 268–9. 2005. doi:10.3322/canjclin.55.5.268
- Hu, Frank (2008). "Interpreting Epidemiologic Evidence and Causal Inference in Obesity Research". In Frank B. Hu. Obesity Epidemiology. New York, NY: Oxford University Press. pp. 38–52. ISBN 0-19-531291-0. Retrieved 2011-02-20
- Omodei, D; Fontana, L (Jun 6, 2011). "Calorie restriction and prevention of age-associated chronic disease". FEBS Lett. 585 (11): 1537–42. PMC 3439843 . PMID 21402069. doi:10.1016/j.febslet.2011.03.015. Retrieved 28 November 2015
- Fontana, L.; Klein, S. (2007). "Aging, Adiposity, and Calorie Restriction". JAMA. 297 (9): 986–94. PMID 17341713. doi:10.1001/jama.297.9.986
- Ghoshal, Kakali (2015). "Adiponectin: Probe of the molecular paradigm associating diabetes and obesity". World Journal of Diabetes. 6 (1): 151–66. PMC 4317307 . PMID 25685286. doi:10.4239/wjd.v6.i1.151
- Heindel, Jerrold (2011). "The Obesogen Hypothesis of Obesity: Overview and Human Evidence". Endocrine updates. 4. 30: 355–365. ISBN 978-1-4419-7033-6. doi:10.1007/978-1-4419-7034-3_17
- Holzman, Donald (2005-05-27). "Panel Suggests Methodology Flawed of Recent CDC Obesity Study". Medscape Medical News. Retrieved 2011-02-21

- Martins, I; Galluzzi, L; Kroemer, G (2011). “Hormesis, cell death and aging”. Aging. 3 (9): 821–8. PMC 3227447. PMID 21931183. doi:10.18632/aging.100380
- Elliott, Sharon; Keim, Nancy L.; Stern, Judith S.; Teff, Karen; Havel, Peter J. (November 2002). “Fructose, weight gain, and the insulin resistance syndrome”. American Journal of Clinical Nutrition. 76 (5): 911–922. PMID 12399260
- Braunwald E (2005). “Chapter 216: heart failure and cor pulmonale”. In Kasper DL, Braunwald E, Fauci AS, et al. Harrison’s Principles of Internal Medicine (16th ed.). New York, NY: McGraw-Hill. pp. 1367–78. ISBN 0-07-139140-1
- Guarente L, Picard F (February 2005). “Calorie Restriction— the SIR2 Connection”. Cell. 120 (4): 473–482. PMID 15734680. doi:10.1016/j.cell.2005.01.029. Retrieved 2015-05-30
- Mattson MP (2005). “Energy intake, meal frequency, and health: a neurobiological perspective”. Annu. Rev. Nutr. (Review). 25: 237–60. PMID 16011467. doi:10.1146/annurev.nutr.25.050304.092526
- Veigas, Nina Maria; Dharmalingam, Mala; Marcus, Sara Rani (2011). “Oxidative Stress in Obesity and Metabolic Syndrome in Asian Indians”. Journal of Medical Biochemistry. 30 (2): 115–20. doi:10.2478/v10011-011-0006-6
- Sizer, Frances Sienkiewicz; Ellie Whitney (2008). Nutrition: Concepts and Controversies (11 ed.). United States of America: Thomson Wadsworth. pp. 221, 235. ISBN 0-495-39065-8
- “Obesity and overweight”. World Health Organization. 2003. Archived from the original on 2011-12-10. Retrieved 2009-04-27
- Piper, Peter W. (2006). “Long-lived yeast as a model for ageing research”. Yeast. 23 (3): 215–26. PMID 16498698. doi:10.1002/yea.1354

3

Nutritional Deficiencies Leading to Malnutrition

Nutritional deficiencies can be of many types like vitamin A deficiency, vitamin E deficiency, vitamin K deficiency and vitamin D deficiency as well as deficiencies which lead to malnutrition such as iodine deficiency, zinc deficiency, hypocalcaemia, mineral deficiency, etc. The aspects elucidated in this section are of vital importance, and provide a better understanding of nutritional deficiencies.

Micronutrient Deficiency

Micronutrient deficiency or dietary deficiency is a lack of one or more of the micronutrients required for plant or animal health. In humans and other animals they include both vitamin deficiencies and mineral deficiencies, whereas in plants the term refers to deficiencies of essential trace minerals.

Humans

Micronutrient deficiencies affect more than two billion people of all ages in both developing and industrialized countries. They are the cause of some diseases, exacerbate others and are recognized as having an important impact on worldwide health. Important micronutrients include iodine, iron, zinc, calcium, selenium, fluorine, and vitamins A, B_6, B_{12}, B_1, B_2, B_3, and C.

Micronutrient deficiencies are associated with 10% of all children's deaths, and are therefore of special concern to those involved with child welfare. Deficiencies of essential vitamins or minerals such as Vitamin A, iron, and zinc may be caused by long-term shortages of nutritious food or by infections such as intestinal worms. They may also be caused or exacerbated when illnesses (such as diarrhoea or malaria) cause rapid loss of nutrients through feces or vomit.

Plants

In plants a micronutrient deficiency (or trace mineral deficiency) is a physiological plant disorder which occurs when a micronutrient is deficient in the soil in which a plant grows. Micronutrients are distinguished from macronutrients (nitrogen, phosphorus, sulfur, potassium, calcium and magnesium) by the relatively low quantities needed by the plant.

A number of elements are known to be needed in these small amounts for proper plant growth and development. Nutrient deficiencies in these areas can adversely affect plant growth and development. Some of the best known trace mineral deficiencies include: zinc deficiency, boron deficiency, iron deficiency, and manganese deficiency.

List of Essential Trace Minerals for Plants

- Boron is believed to be involved in carbohydrate transport in plants; it also assists in metabolic regulation. Boron deficiency will often result in bud dieback.
- Chlorine is necessary for osmosis and ionic balance; it also plays a role in photosynthesis.
- Copper is a component of some enzymes and of vitamin A. Symptoms of copper deficiency include browning of leaf tips and chlorosis.
- Iron is essential for chlorophyll synthesis, which is why an iron deficiency results in chlorosis.
- Manganese activates some important enzymes involved in chlorophyll formation. Manganese deficient plants will develop chlorosis between the veins of its leaves. The availability of manganese is partially dependent on soil pH.
- Molybdenum is essential to plant health. Molybdenum is used by plants to reduce nitrates into usable forms. Some plants use it for nitrogen fixation, thus it may need to be added to some soils before seeding legumes.
- Nickel is essential for activation of urease, an enzyme involved with nitrogen metabolism that is required to process urea.
- Zinc participates in chlorophyll formation, and also activates many enzymes. Symptoms of zinc deficiency include chlorosis and stunted growth.

Vitamin Deficiency

A vitamin deficiency can cause a disease or syndrome known as an avitaminosis or hypovitaminosis. This usually refers to a long-term deficiency of a vitamin. When caused by inadequate nutrition it can be classed as a *primary deficiency*, and when due to an underlying disorder such as malabsorption it can be classed as a *secondary deficiency*. An underlying disorder may be metabolic as in a defect converting tryptophan to niacin. It can also be the result of lifestyle choices including smoking and alcohol consumption.

Examples are vitamin A deficiency, folate deficiency, (scurvy), vitamin D deficiency, vitamin E deficiency, and vitamin K deficiency. In the medical literature, any of these may also be called by names on the pattern of *hypovitaminosis* or *avitaminosis* + *[letter of vitamin]*, for example, hypovitaminosis A, hypovitaminosis C, hypovitaminosis D.

Conversely hypervitaminosis is the syndrome of symptoms caused by over-retention of fat-soluble vitamins in the body.

Types

- Vitamin A is important in growth and development, in the immune system and in eyesight. Its deficiency can cause problems in these areas, particularly in vision; notably night blindness, xerophthalmia and keratomalacia.
- Thiamine (vitamin B1) deficiency can cause beriberi and Wernicke–Korsakoff syndrome.
- Riboflavin deficiency (vitamin B2) causes ariboflavinosis.
- Niacin (vitamin B3) deficiency causes pellagra.
- Pantothenic acid (vitamin B5) deficiency causes chronic paresthesia.
- Biotin (vitamin B7) deficiency negatively affects fertility and hair/skin growth. Deficiency can be caused by poor diet or genetic factors (such as mutations in the BTD gene).
- Folate (vitamin B9) deficiency is associated with numerous health problems. Fortification of certain foods with folate has drastically reduced the incidence of neural tube \effects in countries where such fortification takes place. Deficiency can result from poor diet or genetic factors (such as mutations in the MTHFR gene that lead to compromised folate metabolism).
- Vitamin B12 (cobalamin) deficiency can lead to pernicious anemia, megaloblastic anemia, subacute combined degeneration of spinal cord,and methylmalonic acidemia among other conditions.
- Vitamin C (ascorbic acid) short-term deficiency can lead to weakness, weight loss and general aches and pains. Longer-term depletion may affect the connective tissue. Persistent vitamin C deficiency leads to scurvy.
- Vitamin D (cholecalciferol) deficiency is a known cause of rickets, and has been linked to numerous health problems.
- Vitamin E deficiency causes nerve problems due to poor conduction of electrical impulses along nerves due to changes in nerve membrane structure and function.
- Vitamin K (phylloquinone or menaquinone) deficiency causes impaired coagulation and has also been implicated in osteoporosis.

Vitamin A Deficiency

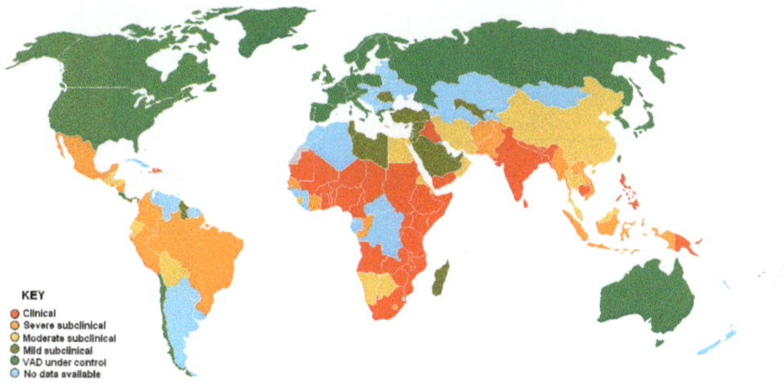

Prevalence of vitamin A deficiency, 1995

Vitamin A deficiency (VAD) or hypovitaminosis A is a lack of vitamin A in blood and tissues. It is common in poorer countries but rarely seen in more developed countries. Nyctalopia (night blindness) is one of the first signs of VAD. Xerophthalmia, keratomalacia, and complete blindness can also occur since Vitamin A has a major role in phototransduction.

Vitamin A deficiency is the leading cause of preventable childhood blindness and is critical to achieving Millennium Development Goal 4 to reduce child mortality. Approximately 250,000 to 500,000 malnourished children in the developing world go blind each year from a deficiency of vitamin A, approximately half of whom die within a year of becoming blind. The United Nations Special Session on Children in 2002 set a goal of the elimination of VAD by 2010.

The prevalence of night blindness due to VAD is also high among pregnant women in many developing countries. VAD also contributes to maternal mortality and other poor outcomes in pregnancy and lactation.

VAD also diminishes the ability to fight infections. In countries where children are not immunized, infectious diseases like measles have higher fatality rates. As elucidated by Alfred Sommer, even mild, subclinical deficiency can also be a problem, as it may increase children's risk of developing respiratory and diarrheal infections, decrease growth rate, slow bone development, and decrease likelihood of survival from serious illness.

VAD is estimated to affect approximately one third of children under the age of five around the world. It is estimated to claim the lives of 670,000 children under five annually. Approximately 250,000–500,000 children in developing countries become blind each year owing to VAD, with the highest prevalence in Southeast Asia and Africa. According to the World Health Organization (WHO), VAD is under control in the United States, but, in developing countries, VAD is a significant concern. Globally, 65% of all children aged 6 to 59 months received two doses of vitamin A in 2013, fully protecting them against VAD (80% in the least developed countries).

Signs and Symptoms

The common cause of blindness in developing countries is VAD. The World Health Organization (WHO) estimates 13.8 million children to have some degree of visual loss related to VAD. Night blindness and its worsened condition, xerophthalmia, are markers of VAD, as it can also lead to impaired immune function, cancer, and birth defects. Collections of keratin in the conjunctiva, known as Bitot's spots, are also seen. Imtiaz's sign is the earliest ocular sign of VAD. Conjunctival epithelial defects occur around lateral aspect of the limbus in subclinical stage of VAD. These conjunctival epithelial defects are not even visible on a biomicroscope, but they take up black stain and become readily visible after instillation of kajal (surma); this is called "Imtiaz's sign".

Night blindness is the difficulty for the eyes to adjust to dim light. Affected individuals are unable to distinguish images in low levels of illumination. People with night blindness have poor vision in the darkness, but see normally when adequate light is present.

VAD affects vision by inhibiting the production of rhodopsin, the eye pigment responsible for sensing low light situations. Rhodopsin is found in the retina and is composed of retinal (an active form of vitamin A) and opsin (a protein). Because the body cannot create retinal in sufficient amounts, a diet low in vitamin A will lead to a decreased amount of rhodopsin in the eye, as there is inadequate retinal to bind with opsin. Night blindness results.

Night blindness caused by VAD has been associated with the loss of goblet cells in the conjunctiva, a membrane covering the outer surface of the eye. Goblet cells are responsible for secretion of mucus, and their absence results in xerophthalmia, a condition where the eyes fail to produce tears. Dead epithelial and microbial cells accumulate on the conjunctiva and form debris that can lead to infection and possibly blindness.

Decreasing night blindness requires the improvement of vitamin A status in at-risk populations. Supplements and fortification of food have been shown to be effective interventions. Supplement treatment for night blindness includes high doses of vitamin A (200,000 IU) in the form of retinyl palmitate to be taken by mouth, which is administered two to four times a year. Intramuscular injections are poorly absorbed and are ineffective in delivering sufficient bio-available vitamin A. Fortification of food with vitamin A is costly, but can be done in wheat, sugar, and milk. Households may circumvent expensive fortified food by altering dietary habits. Consumption of yellow-orange fruits and vegetables rich in carotenoids, specifically beta-carotene, provides pro-vitamin A precursors that can prevent VAD related night blindness. However, the conversion of carotene to retinol varies from person to person and bioavailability of carotene in food varies.

The richest animal sources of Vitamin A (retinol) are livers like beef liver (one ounce provides around 8,000 IUs) and Cod Liver Oil (one teaspoon provides around 4,500 IUs).

Vitamin A deficiency is one of several hypovitaminoses implicated in follicular hyperkeratosis.

Causes

The major cause is roughage which include few animal sources of pre-formed vitamin A. In addition to dietary problems, there are other causes of VAD. Iron deficiency can affect vitamin A uptake. Excess alcohol consumption can deplete vitamin A, and a stressed liver may be more susceptible to vitamin A toxicity. People who consume large amounts of alcohol should seek medical advice before taking vitamin A supplements. In general, people should also seek medical advice before taking vitamin A supplements if they have any condition associated with fat malabsorption such as pancreatitis, cystic fibrosis, tropical sprue and biliary obstruction. Other causes of Vitamin A deficiency are inadequate intake, fat malabsorption, or liver disorders. Deficiency impairs immunity and hematopoiesis and causes rashes and typical ocular effects (e.g., xerophthalmia, night blindness).

Infection Rates

Along with poor diet there is a large amount of infection and disease present in many developing communities. Infection is very draining on vitamin A reserves and this vitamin A deficit leaves the individual more susceptible to infection (Combs, 1991); increased documentation of xerophthalmia has been seen after an outbreak of measles and the varying stages of xerophthalmia become a good reference point for the extent of deficiency (with mortality increasing with severity of the eye disease). In a longitudinal study of preschool Indonesian children it was found that susceptibility to disease increased nine times when severe VAD was present (Dole 2009).

The reason for the increased infection rate in vitamin A deficient populations is due to the T-killer cells which require retinoids to proliferate correctly (Athanassiades1981). Retinoic acid binds the promoter region of specific genes and so activates the transcription process and therefore cell replication (Baron 1981). A vitamin A deficient diet will have a very limited surplus of retinol and so cell proliferation and replication will be suppressed, contributing to a reduced number of T-cells and lymphocytes. Suppression of these will result in a lack of immune reaction if pathogens become present in the body and consequently a greater susceptibility to incubation of disease.

VAD and infections aggravate each other and therefore with infection the vitamin A levels are depleted which in turn reduces intestinal absorption of vitamin A (WHO 1982). Very often seen with VAD is protein energy malnutrition (PEM). With PEM the synthesis of retinol binding protein (RBP) is decreased, consequently the uptake of retinol is reduced (Combs, 1991). This leads to an inability to utilise any vitamin A present as the RBP is absent and so the retinol cannot be transported to the liver maximising the VAD (Ikekpeazu 2010).

Treatment

Treatment of VAD can be undertaken with both oral and injectable forms, generally as vitamin A palmitate.

- As an oral form, the supplementation of vitamin A is effective for lowering the risk of morbidity, especially from severe diarrhea, and reducing mortality from measles and all-cause mortality. Studies have shown that vitamin A supplementation of children under five who are at risk of VAD can reduce all-cause mortality by 23 per cent. Some countries where VAD is a public health problem address its elimination by including vitamin A supplements available in capsule form with National Immunization Days (NIDs) for polio eradication or measles. Additionally, the delivery of vitamin A supplements, during integrated child health events such as child health days, have helped ensure high coverage of vitamin A supplementation in a large number of least developed countries. Child health events enable many countries in West and Central Africa to achieve over 80 per cent coverage of vitamin A supplementation. According to UNICEF Data, in 2013 worldwide, 65 per cent of children between the ages of 6 and 59 months were fully protected with two high-dose vitamin A supplements. Vitamin A capsules cost about US$0.02. The capsules are easy to handle; they don't need to be stored in a refrigerator or vaccine carrier. When the correct dosage is given, vitamin A is safe and has no negative effect on seroconversion rates for Oral Polio Vaccine or measles vaccine. However, because the benefit of vitamin A supplements is transient, children need them regularly every four to six months. Since NIDs provide only one dose per year, NIDs-linked vitamin A distribution must be complemented by other dose programs to maintain vitamin A in children Maternal high supplementation benefits both mother and breast-fed infant: high-dose vitamin A supplementation of the lactating mother in the first month postpartum can provide the breast-fed infant with an appropriate amount of vitamin A through breast milk. However, high-dose supplementation of pregnant women should be avoided because it can cause miscarriage and birth defects.

- Food fortification is also useful for improving VAD. A variety of oily and dry forms of the retinol esters, retinyl acetates and retinyl palmitate are available for food fortification of vitamin A. Margarine and oil are the ideal food vehicles for vitamin A fortification. They protect vitamin A from oxidation during storage and prompt absorption of vitamin A. Beta-carotene and retinyl acetate or retinyl palmitate are used as a form of vitamin A for vitamin A fortification of fat-based foods. Fortification of sugar with retinyl palmitate as a form of vitamin A has been used extensively throughout Central America. Cereal flours, milk powder, and liquid milk are also used as food vehicles for vitamin A fortification. Genetic engineering is another method of food fortification, and this has been achieved with golden rice, but opposition to genetically modified foods has prevented its use as of July 2012.

- Dietary diversification can also control VAD. Non-animal sources of vitamin A which contain pre-formed vitamin A account for greater than 80% of intake for most individuals in the developing world. The increase in consumption of vitamin A-rich foods of animal origin in addition to fruits and vegetables has beneficial effects on VAD. Researchers at the Agricultural Research Service have been able to identify genetic sequences in corn that are associated with higher levels of beta-carotene, the precursor to vitamin A. They found that breeders can cross certain variations of corn to produce a crop with an 18-fold increase in beta-carotene. Such advancements in nutritional plant breeding could one day aid in the illnesses related to VAD in developing countries.

Global Initiatives

Global efforts to support national governments in addressing VAD are led by the Global Alliance for Vitamin A (GAVA), which is an informal partnership between A2Z, the Canadian International Development Agency, Helen Keller International, Micronutrient Initiative, UNICEF, USAID, and the World Bank. Joint GAVA activity is coordinated by the Micronutrient Initiative.

Vitamin Angels has committed itself to eradicating childhood blindness due to VAD on the planet by the year 2020. Operation 20/20 was launched in 2007 and will cover 18 countries. The program gives children two high-dose vitamin A and anti-parasitic supplements (twice a year for four years), which provides children with enough of the nutrient during their most vulnerable years in order to prevent them from going blind and suffering from other life-threatening diseases caused by VAD.

About 75 per cent of the vitamin A required for supplementation activity by developing countries is supplied by the Micronutrient Initiative with support from the Canadian International Development Agency.

An estimated 1.25 million deaths due to VAD have been averted in 40 countries since 1998.

In 2008 it was estimated that an annual investment of US$60 million in vitamin A and zinc supplementation combined would yield benefits of more than US$1 billion per year, with every dollar spent generating benefits of more than US$17. These combined interventions were ranked by the Copenhagen Consensus 2008 as the world's best development investment.

Epidemiology

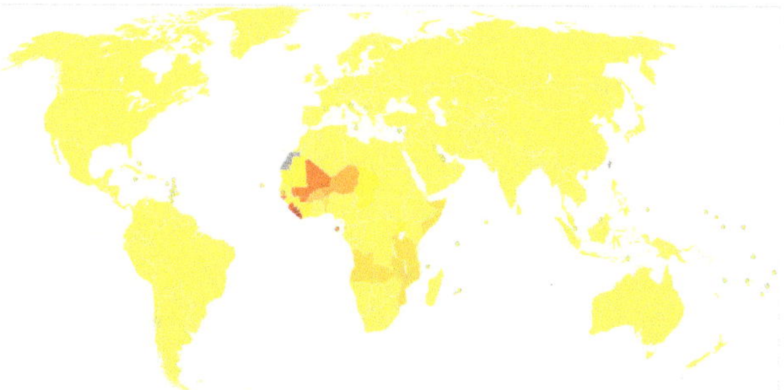

Disability-adjusted life year for vitamin A deficiency per 100,000 inhabitants in 2002.

no data	105–140	245–280
less than 35	140–175	280–315
35–70	175–210	315–350
70–105	210–245	350–400
		more than 400

Vitamin D Deficiency

Vitamin D deficiency, or hypovitaminosis D, can result from inadequate nutritional intake of vitamin D, inadequate sunlight exposure (in particular sunlight with adequate ultraviolet B rays), disorders limiting vitamin D absorption, and conditions impairing vitamin D conversion into active metabolites—including certain liver, kidney, and hereditary disorders. Deficiency impairs bone mineralization, leading to bone softening diseases as rickets in children and osteomalacia and osteoporosis in adults.

Classifications

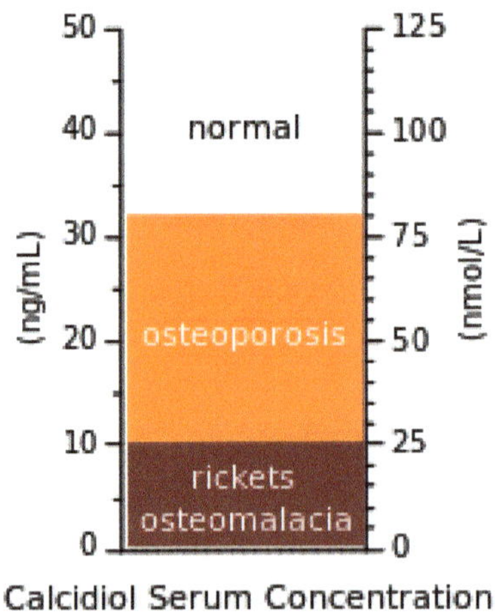

Mapping of several bone diseases onto levels of vitamin D (calcidiol) in the blood

Vitamin D deficiency is typically diagnosed by measuring the concentration of the prehormone calcidiol (25-hydroxyvitamin D) in the blood. which is a precursor to the active form 1,25-dihydroxyvitamin D (calcitriol). One 2008 review has proposed the following categories for hypovitaminosis D:

- Insufficient 25–74 nmol/L (10–29.6 ng/mL)
- Normal Range 75–250 nmol/L

These ranges are based on a Canadian range. Season, race and dietary intake affect 25-HydroxyVitamin D levels. Highest levels are found in the summer months and lowest levels during the winter. Other authors have also suggested that a 25-hydroxyvitamin D level of 75–80 nmol/L (30–32 ng/mL) may be sufficient although a majority of healthy young people with comparatively extreme sun exposure did not reach this level in a study done in Hawaii.

Note that 1.0 nmol/L = 0.4 ng/mL for this compound.

Signs and Symptoms

Vitamin D deficiency is known to cause several problems, including:

- It has found to be associated with the advancement of cancers, for example; breast, colon, ovarian, and prostate.
- Depression (discussed below)
- Increased risk of fracture- In an elderly population, the incidence of nonvertebral fractures was reduced between 32 and 68% as an effect of vitamin D being supplemented.
- Light-headedness
- Muscle aches and weakness (in particular the limb girdles)
- Muscle twitching (fasciculations) is commonly seen due to reduced ionised calcium, arising from a low vitamin D.
- Osteomalacia, a bone-thinning disorder that occurs exclusively in adults and is characterized by proximal muscle weakness and bone fragility.
- Osteoporosis, a condition characterized by reduced bone mineral density and increased bone fragility.
- Periodontitis, local inflammatory bone loss that can result in tooth loss
- Rickets, a childhood disease characterized by impeded growth and deformity of the long bones. The earliest sign of subclinical vitamin D deficiency is craniotabes, abnormal softening or thinning of the skull.

The role of diet in the development of rickets was determined by Edward Mellanby between 1918 and 1920. In 1921, Elmer McCollum identified an antirachitic substance found in certain fats that could prevent rickets. Because the newly discovered substance was the fourth vitamin identified, it was called vitamin D. The 1928 Nobel Prize in Chemistry was awarded to Adolf Windaus, who discovered the steroid 7-dehydrocholesterol, the precursor of vitamin D.

Prior to the fortification of milk products with vitamin D, rickets was a major public health problem. In the United States, milk has been fortified with 10 micrograms (400 IU) of vitamin D per quart since the 1930s, leading to a dramatic decline in the number of rickets cases. Vitamin D deficiency can be asymptomatic, but may also affect bone mineralization, resulting in failure to achieve an optimal peak bone mass, which increases fracture risk in both childhood and adult life.

Risk Factors

Those most likely to be affected by vitamin D deficiency are people with little or no solar exposure. Climate, dress habits, avoiding sun exposure and too much sunscreen protection limit the production of vitamin D.

Age

The amount of vitamin D recommended for all infants, children, and adolescents has recently increased – from 400 to 600 IU per day. The National Academy of Medicine (NAM) released the Consensus Report on Dietary Reference Intakes for Calcium and Vitamin D on November 30, 2010. The recommendation was for 600 IU of vitamin D a day for those 1-70 and 800 IU for those over 70 years of age. As of October 2008, the American Pediatric Association advises vitamin D supplementation of 400 IU/day (10 μg/d) from birth onwards. (1 IU vitamin D is the biological equivalent of 0.025 μg cholecalciferol/ergocalciferol.) The daily dose of 400 IU is required to prevent rickets and possibly also a wide range of chronic nonskeletal diseases. The Canadian Paediatric Society recommends that pregnant or breastfeeding women consider taking 2000 IU/day, that all babies who are exclusively breastfed receive a supplement of 400 IU/day, and that babies living north of 55°N get 800 IU/day from October to April. Health Canada recommends 400IU/day (10 μg/d). Infant formula is generally fortified with vitamin D. Hypovitaminosis D is common in postmenopausal women, regardless of whether they are healthy or have other medical conditions.

Malnutrition

Although rickets and osteomalacia are now rare in Britain, osteomalacia outbreaks in some immigrant communities included women with seemingly adequate daylight outdoor exposure wearing Western clothing. Having darker skin and reduced exposure to sunshine did not produce rickets unless the diet deviated from a Western omnivore pattern characterized by high intakes of meat, fish, and eggs, and low intakes of high-extraction cereals. The dietary risk factors for rickets include abstaining from animal foods. Vitamin D deficiency remains the main cause of rickets among young infants in most countries, because breast milk is low in vitamin D and social customs and climatic conditions can prevent adequate UVB exposure. In sunny countries, such as Nigeria, South Africa, and Bangladesh, where the disease occurs among older toddlers and children, it has been attributed to low dietary calcium intakes, which are characteristic of cereal-based diets with limited access to dairy products. Rickets was formerly a major public health problem among the US population; in Denver, where ultraviolet rays are about 20% stronger than at sea level on the same latitude, almost two-thirds of 500 children had mild rickets in the late 1920s. An increase in the proportion of animal protein in the 20th-century American diet coupled with increased consumption of milk fortified with relatively small quantities of vitamin D coincided with a dramatic decline in the number of rickets cases.

Obesity

Obese individuals have lower levels of the circulating form of vitamin D, due to the likelihood of decreased bioavailability of vitamin D_3 from food and sunlight due to the distribution in adipose tissue. A population-based cohort study in Spain tested 1226 subjects to determine the connection between obesity and hypovitaminosis D; the study reported, "vitamin D deficiency is associated with an increase risk of developing obesity."

Sun Exposure

The use of sunscreen with a sun protection factor of 8 can theoretically inhibit more than 95% of vitamin D production in the skin. In practice, however, sunscreen is applied so as to have a negligible effect on vitamin D status. The vitamin D status of those in Australia and New Zealand is unlikely to have been affected by campaigns advocating sunscreen. Instead, wearing clothing is more effective at reducing the amount of skin exposed to UVB and reducing natural vitamin D synthesis. Clothing which covers a large portion of the skin, when worn on a consistent and regular basis, such as the burqa, is correlated with lower vitamin D levels and an increased prevalence of hypovitaminosis D.

Regions far from the equator have a high seasonal variation of the amount and intensity of sunlight. In the UK the prevalence of low vitamin D status in children and adolescents is found to be higher in winter than in summer. Lifestyle factors such as indoor versus outdoor work and time spent in outdoor recreation play an important role.

Habitation and Living Conditions

Hypovitaminosis D has been associated with urbanisation in terms of both air pollution, which blocks UV light, and an increase in the number of people working indoors. The elderly are generally exposed to less UV light due to hospitalisation, immobility, institutionalisation, and being housebound, leading to decreased levels of vitamin D.

Darker Skin Color

The reduced pigmentation of light-skinned individuals may result in higher vitamin D levels and that, because melanin acts like a sun-block, dark-skinned individuals, in particular, may require extra vitamin D to avoid deficiency at higher latitudes. Sub-Saharan African people are at a higher risk to be vitamin deficient due to their skin color and the melanin levels. The natural selection hypothesis suggests that lighter skin color evolved to optimise vitamin D production in extreme northern and southern latitudes.

Malabsorption

Rates of vitamin D deficiency are higher among people with untreated celiac disease, inflammatory bowel disease, exocrine pancreatic insufficiency from cystic fibrosis, and short bowel syndrome, which can all produce problems of malabsorption.

Critical Illness

Vitamin D deficiency is relatively common in the general population, amounting to an incidence of 82% in critically ill patients. Vitamin D deficiency is associated with increased mortality in critical illness. People who take vitamin D supplements before being admitted for intensive care are less likely to die than those who do not take vitamin D supplements. Additionally, vitamin D levels decline during stays in intensive care.

A 2016 systematic review and meta-analysis of the relationship between vitamin D and mortality in critical illness showed that vitamin D3 (cholecalciferol) or calcitriol given orally can reduce mortality rate without significant adverse effects.

Pathophysiology

Vitamin D deficiency leads to impaired intestinal absorption of calcium, which results in decreased levels of serum total and ionized calcium levels. This hypocalcemia gives rise to secondary hyperparathyroidism, which is a homeostatic response aimed at maintaining, initially, serum calcium levels at the expense of the skeleton. Following this parathyroid hormone-induced increase in bone turnover, alkaline phosphatase levels are often increased. PTH not only increases bone resorption, but also leads to decreased urinary calcium excretion while promoting phosphaturia. This results in hypophosphatemia, which exacerbates the mineralization defect in the skeleton.

Diagnosis

The serum concentration of 25(OH)D is typically used to determine vitamin D status. It reflects vitamin D produced in the skin, as well as that acquired from the diet, and has a fairly long circulating half-life of 15 days. It does not, however, reveal the amount of vitamin D stored in other body tissues.

The level of serum 1,25(OH)D is not usually used to determine vitamin D status because it has a short half-life of 15 hours and is tightly regulated by parathyroid hormone, calcium, and phosphate, such that it does not decrease significantly until vitamin D deficiency is already well advanced.

Variability in results of laboratory analyses of the level of 25(OH)D occurs. Falsely low or high values have been obtained depending on the particular test or laboratory used. Beginning in July 2009, a standard reference material became available which should allow laboratories to standardise their procedures.

Some disagreement exists concerning the exact levels of 25(OH)D needed for good health. A level lower than 10 ng/mL (25 nmol/L) is associated with the most severe deficiency diseases: rickets in infants and children, and osteomalacia in adults. A concentration above 15 ng/ml (37.5 nmol/L) is generally considered adequate for those in good health. Levels above 30 ng/ml (75 nmol/L) are proposed by some as desirable for achieving optimum health, but not yet enough evidence exists to support this.

Levels of 25(OH)D that are consistently above 200 ng/mL (500 nmol/L) are thought to be potentially toxic, although data from humans are sparse. In animal studies, levels up to 400 ng/mL (1,000 nmol/L) were not associated with toxicity. Vitamin D toxicity usually results from taking supplements in excess. Hypercalcemia is typically the cause of symptoms, and levels of 25(OH)D above 150 ng/mL (375 nmol/L) are usually found, although in some cases 25(OH)D levels may appear to be normal. Periodic measurement of serum calcium in individuals receiving large doses of vitamin D is recommended.

In overweight persons, increased fat mass is inversely associated with 25(OH)D levels. This association may confound the reported relationships between low vitamin D status and conditions which occur more commonly in obesity as the circulating 25(OH) D underestimates their total body stores. However, as vitamin D is fat-soluble, excess amounts can be stored in fat tissue and used during winter, when sun exposure is limited.

A study of highly sun-exposed (tanned) healthy young skateboarders and surfers in Hawaii found levels below the proposed higher minimum of 30 ng/ml in 51% of the subjects. The highest 25(OH)D concentration was around 60 ng/ml (150nmol/L). A similar <using the same data>study in Hawaii found a range of (11–71 ng/mL) in a population with prolonged extensive skin exposure, while as part of the same study Wisconsin breastfeeding mothers were given supplements. The range of circulating 25(OH)D levels in women in the supplementated group was from 12–77 ng/mL. Levels in the supplemented population in Wisconsin were higher than the sun-exposed group in Hawaii (which again included surfers because it was the same data set).

Another study of African Americans found that blood levels of 25(OH)D decreased linearly with increasing African ancestry, the decrease being 2.5-2.75 nmol/L per 10% increase in African ancestry. Sunlight and diet were 46% less effective in raising these levels among subjects with high African ancestry than among those with low/medium African ancestry. Vitamin-D metabolism possibly differs by ethnicity.

Skin colour has been associated with low 25(OH)D, especially in Africans living in countries with a temperate climate. For example, 25-OHD under 10 ng/mL (25 nmol/l) in 44% of asymptomatic East African children living in Melbourne A study of healthy young Ethiopians living in Addis Ababa (10 degrees N) found average 25(OH)D levels of 23.5nmol/L. A review of vitamin D in Africa gives the median levels for equatorial countries: Kenya 65.5 nmol/L and Democratic Republic of the Congo 65nmol/L, concluding that it remains to be established if associations between vitamin D status and health outcomes identified in Western countries can be replicated in African countries.

Vitamin D levels are around 30% higher in northern Europe than in central and southern Europe; higher vitamin D concentrations in northern countries may have a genetic basis. In a meta-analysis of cross-sectional studies on serum 25(OH)D concentrations globally, the levels averaged 54 nmol/l and were higher in women than men, and higher in Caucasians than in non-Caucasians. No trend in serum 25(OH)D level was related to latitude. African Americans often have a very low circulating 25(OH)D level. However, those of African descent have higher parathyroid hormone and 1,25-Dihydroxycholecalciferol associated with lower 25-hydroxyvitamin D than other ethnic groups; moreover, they have the greatest bone density and lowest risk of fragility fractures compared to other populations.

Rickets is sometimes due to genetic disorders such as autosomal dominant hypophosphatemic rickets or X-linked hypophosphatemia and associated with consanguineous marriage, and possibly founder effect. In Kashmir, India patients with pseudovitamin D deficiency rickets had grossly raised 25-hydroxyvitamin D concentrations.

Screening

The usefulness of screening adults without symptoms of vitamin D deficiency is unclear.

Treatment

The replacement of vitamin D needs for treating Vitamin D deficiency depends on the severity of the deficiency. Treatment involves an initial high-dosage treatment phase until the required serum levels are reached, followed by the maintenance of the acquired levels. The lower the 25(OH)D serum concentration is before treatment, the higher is the dosage that is needed in order to quickly reach an acceptable serum level.

The initial high-dosage treatment can be given on a daily or weekly basis or can be given in form of one or several single doses (also known as *stoss therapy*, from the German word "Stoß" meaning *push*).

Therapy prescriptions vary, and there is no consensus yet on how best to arrive at an optimum serum level. While per mole vitamin D_3 is more potent to raise 25(OH)D blood levels than vitamin D_2, per IU both D_2 and D_3 are equal for maintaining 25(OH) D status.

Initial Phase

Daily or Weekly Dose

For treating rickets, the American Academy of Pediatrics (AAP) has recommended that pediatric patients receive an initial two- to three-month treatment of "high-dose" vitamin D therapy. In this regime, the daily dosis of cholecalciferol is 1,000 IU for newborns, 1,000 to 5,000 IU for 1- to 12-months old infants, and 5,000 IU for patients over 1 year of age.

For adults, other dosages have been called for. A review of 2008/2009 recommended dosages of 1,000 IU cholecalciferol per 10 nmol/l required serum increase, to be given daily over two to three months. In another proposed cholecalciferol loading dose guideline for vitamin D-deficient adults, a weekly dosage is given, up to a total amount that is proportional to the required serum increase (up to the level of 75 nml/l) and, within certain body weight limits, to body weight.

Single-dose Therapy

Alternatively, a single-dose therapy is used for instance if there are concerns regarding the patient's compliance. The single-dose therapy can be given as an injection, but is normally given in form of an oral medication.

Maintenance Phase

Once the desired serum levels has been achieved, be it by a high daily or weekly dose or by a single-dose therapy, the AAP recommendation calls for a maintenance supplementation of 400 IU for all age groups, with this dosage being doubled for premature infants, dark-skinned infants and children, children who reside in areas of limited sun exposure (>37.5° latitude), obese patients, and those on certain medications.

Special Cases

To maintain blood levels of calcium, therapeutic vitamin D doses are sometimes administered (up to 100,000 IU or 2.5 mg daily) to patients who have had their parathyroid glands removed (most commonly kidney dialysis patients who have had tertiary hyperparathyroidism, but also to patients with primary hyperparathyroidism) or with hypoparathyroidism. Patients with chronic liver disease or intestinal malabsorption disorders may also require larger doses of vitamin D (up to 40,000 IU or 1 mg (1000 micrograms) daily).

Epidemiology

The estimated percentage of the population with a vitamin D deficiency varies based on the threshold used to define a deficiency.

Percentage of U.S. population	Definition of insufficiency	Study
69.5%	25(OH)D less than 30 ng/mL	Chowdury *et al.* 2014
77%	25(OH)D less than 30 ng/mL	Ginde *et al.* 2009
36%	25(OH)D less than 20 ng/mL	Ginde *et al.* 2009
6%	25(OH)D less than 10 ng/mL	Ginde *et al.* 2009

Recommendations for 25(OH)D serum levels vary across authorities, and probably vary based on factors like age; calculations for the epidemiology of vitamin D deficiency depend on the recommended level used.

A 2011 Institute of Medicine report set the sufficiency level at 20 ng/ml (50 nmol/l), while in the same year The Endocrine Society defined sufficient serum levels at 30 ng/ml and others have set the level as high as 60 ng/ml. As of 2011 most reference labs used the 30 ng/ml standard.

Applying the IOM standard to NHANES data on serum levels, for the period from 1988 to 1994 22% of the US population was deficient, and 36% were deficient for the period between 2001 and 2004; applying the Endocrine Society standard, 55% of the US population was deficient between 1988 and 1994, and 77% were deficient for the period between 2001 and 2004.

In 2011 the Centers for Disease Control and Prevention applied the IOM standard to NHANES data on serum levels collected between 2001 and 2006, and determined that 32% of Americans were deficient during that period (8% at risk of deficiency, and 24% at risk of inadequacy).

Research

A great deal of research has been conducted to understand whether low levels of vitamin D may cause, or be caused by, other conditions.

Vitamin D deficiency is thought to play a role in the pathogenesis of non-alcoholic fatty liver disease.

Hypovitaminosis D is a risk factor for depression; some studies have found that low levels of vitamin D are correlated with depressed feelings and are found in patients who have been diagnosed with depression. Hypovitaminosis D is linked to the development and severity of depression

Some evidence suggests hypovitaminosis D may be associated with a worse outcome for some cancers, but evidence is insufficient to recommend that vitamin D be prescribed for people with cancer. Taking vitamin D supplements has no significant effect on cancer risk. Vitamin D_3, however, appears to decrease the risk of death from cancer but concerns with the quality of the data exist.

Vitamin D deficiency is correlated with the development of pre-eclampsia in pregnancy. Maternal vitamin D deficiency may affect the baby, causing overt bone disease from before birth and impairment of bone quality after birth.

Vitamin E Deficiency

Vitamin E deficiency or hypovitaminosis E is a deficiency of vitamin E. It causes nerve problems due to poor conduction of electrical impulses along nerves due to changes in nerve membrane structure and function.

Signs and Symptoms

Signs of vitamin E deficiency include the following:

- Neuromuscular problems-such as spinocerebellar ataxia and myopathies.
- Neurological problems-may include dysarthria, absence of deep tendon reflexes, loss of vibratory sensation and proprioception, and positive Babinski sign.
- Anemia-due to oxidative damage to red blood cells
- Retinopathy
- Impairment of the immune response

There is also some laboratory evidence that vitamin E deficiency can cause male infertility.

Causes

Vitamin E deficiency is rare and is almost never caused by a poor diet. Instead, there are three specific situations when a vitamin E deficiency is likely to occur:

- Premature, very low birth weight infants - birth weights less than 1500 grams, or 3.5 pounds. A neonatologist, a pediatrician specializing in the care of newborns, typically evaluates the nutritional needs of premature infants.
- Rare disorders of fat metabolism - There is a rare genetic condition termed isolated vitamin E deficiency or 'ataxia with isolated with vitamin E deficiency', caused by mutations in the gene for the tocopherol transfer protein. These individuals have an extremely poor capacity to absorb vitamin E and develop neurological complications that are reversed by high doses of vitamin E.
- Fat malabsorption - Some dietary fat is needed for the absorption of vitamin E from the gastrointestinal tract. Anyone diagnosed with cystic fibrosis, individuals who have had part or all of their stomach removed or who have had a gastric bypass, and individuals with malabsorptive problems such as Crohn's disease, liver disease or pancreatic insufficiency may not absorb fat (people who cannot absorb fat often pass greasy stools or have chronic diarrhea and bloating). Abetalipoproteinemia is a rare inherited disorder of fat metabolism that results in poor absorption of dietary fat and vitamin E. The vitamin E deficiency associated with this disease causes problems such as poor transmission of nerve impulses, muscle weakness, and degeneration of the retina that can cause blindness.

Mechanism

- Visual changes-Photoreceptor outer segment membranes have a very high concentration of polyunsaturated fatty acids (PUFA's) and are potentially very susceptible to oxidative damage (the retina consumes 5-10 times more oxygen per milligram than any other tissue tested). Vitamin E is present in the outer segment and is the only well-recognized chain-breaking, lipid-soluble antioxidant in vivo. After 12 months of experimental vitamin E deficiency in rats, visual function was absent or grossly abnormal. There was a 90% loss of DHA from the retina-probably caused by peroxidative degradation-and changes in retinal membrane fluidity.

Treatment

The treatment is some form of Vitamin E supplementation.

Aggressive vitamin E replacement therapy has been shown to either prevent, halt or improve visual abnormalities.

Vitamin K Deficiency

Vitamin K deficiency or hypovitaminosis K is a form of avitaminosis resulting from insufficient vitamin K_1 or vitamin K_2 or both.

Signs and Symptoms

Symptoms include bruising, petechiae, hematomas, oozing of blood at surgical or puncture sites, stomach pains; risk of massive uncontrolled bleeding; cartilage calcification; and severe malformation of developing bone or deposition of insoluble calcium salts in the walls of arteries. In infants, it can cause some birth defects such as underdeveloped face, nose, bones, and fingers.

Vitamin K is changed to its active form in the liver by the enzyme Vitamin K epoxide reductase. Activated vitamin K is then used to gamma carboxylate (and thus activate) certain enzymes involved in coagulation: Factors II, VII, IX, X, and protein C and protein S. Inability to activate the clotting cascade via these factors leads to the bleeding symptoms mentioned above.

Notably, when one examines the lab values in Vitamin K deficiency the prothrombin time is elevated, but the partial thromboplastin time is normal or only mildly prolonged. This may seem counterintuitive given that the deficiency leads to decreased activity in factors of both the intrinsic pathway (F-IX) which is monitored by PTT, as well as the extrinsic pathway (F-VII) which is monitored by PT. However, factor VII has the shortest half-life of all the factors carboxylated by vitamin K; therefore, when deficient, it is the PT that rises first, since the activated Factor VII is the first to "disappear." In later stages of deficiency, the other factors (which have longer half lives) are able to "catch up," and the PTT becomes elevated as well.

Cause

Vitamin K_1-deficiency may occur by disturbed intestinal uptake (such as would occur in a bile duct obstruction), by therapeutic or accidental intake of a vitamin K_1-antagonist such as warfarin, or, very rarely, by nutritional vitamin K_1 deficiency. As a result, Gla-residues are inadequately formed and the Gla-proteins are insufficiently active.

Treatment

Vitamin K_2 Deficiency

Menaquinone (vitamin K_2), but not phylloquinone (vitamin K_1), intake is associated with reduced risk of CHD mortality, all-cause mortality and severe aortic calcification.

Epidemiology

The prevalence of vitamin K deficiency varies by geographic region. For infants in the United States, vitamin K_1 deficiency without bleeding may occur in as many as 50% of infants younger than 5 days old, with the classic hemorrhagic disease occurring in 0.25-1.7% of infants. Therefore, the Committee on Nutrition of the American Academy of Pediatrics recommends that 0.5 to 1.0 mg Vitamin K_1 be administered to all newborns shortly after birth.

Postmenopausal and elderly women in Thailand have high risk of Vitamin K_2 deficiency, compared with the normal value of young, reproductive females. Current dosage recommendations for Vitamin K may be too low. The deposition of calcium in soft tissues, including arterial walls, is quite common, especially in those suffering from atherosclerosis, suggesting that Vitamin K deficiency is more common than previously thought.

Because colonic bacteria synthesize a significant portion of the Vitamin K required for human needs, individuals with disruptions to or insufficient amounts of these bacteria can be at risk for Vitamin K deficiency. Newborns, as mentioned above, fit into this category, as their colons are frequently not adequately colonized in the first five to seven days of life. (Consumption of the mother's milk can undo this temporary problem.) Another at-risk population comprises those individuals on any sort of long-term antibiotic therapy, as this can diminish the population of normal gut flora.

B Vitamins

B vitamins are a class of water-soluble vitamins that play important roles in cell metabolism. Though these vitamins share similar names, research shows that they are chemically distinct vitamins that often coexist in the same foods. In general, dietary supplements containing all eight are referred to as a vitamin B complex. Individual B vitamin supplements are referred to by the specific name of each vitamin (e.g. B_1, B_2, B_3 etc.).

Riboflavin

Riboflavin, also known as vitamin B_2, is a vitamin found in food and used as a dietary supplement. As a supplement it is used to prevent and treat riboflavin deficiency and prevent migraines. It may be given by mouth or injection.

It is nearly always well tolerated. Normal doses are safe during pregnancy. Riboflavin is in the vitamin B group. It is required by the body for cellular respiration. Food sources include eggs, green vegetables, milk, and meat.

Riboflavin was discovered in 1920, isolated in 1933, and first made in 1935. It is on the World Health Organization's List of Essential Medicines, the most effective and safe medicines needed in a health system. Riboflavin is available as a generic medication and over the counter. In the United States a month of supplements costs less than 25 USD. Some countries require its addition to grains.

Medical Uses

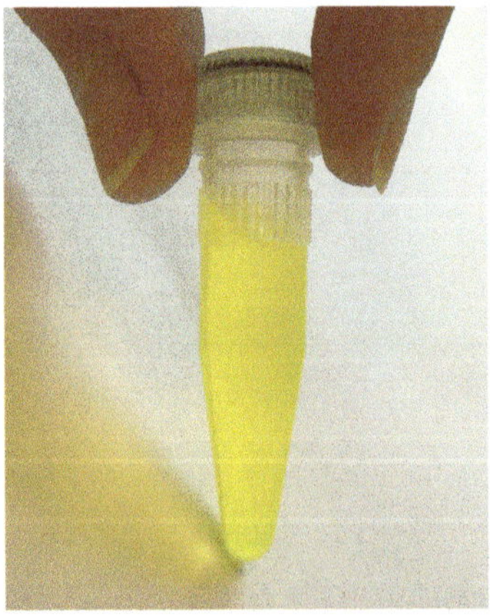

A solution of riboflavin.

Riboflavin has been used in several clinical and therapeutic situations. For over 30 years, riboflavin supplements have been used as part of the phototherapy treatment of neonatal jaundice. The light used to irradiate the infants breaks down not only bilirubin, the toxin causing the jaundice, but also the naturally occurring riboflavin within the infant's blood, so extra supplementation is necessary.

One clinical trial found that high-dose riboflavin appears to be useful alone or along with beta-blockers in the prevention of migraine. A dose of 400 mg daily has been used effectively in the prophylaxis of migraines, especially in combination with a daily supplement of magnesium citrate 500 mg and, in some cases, a supplement of coenzyme Q10. However, two other clinical studies have failed to find any significant results for the effectiveness of B2 as a treatment for migraine.

Riboflavin in combination with UV light has been shown to be effective in reducing the ability of harmful pathogens found in blood products to cause disease. When UV light is applied to blood products containing riboflavin, the nucleic acids in pathogens are damaged, rendering them unable to replicate and cause disease. Riboflavin and UV light treatment has been shown to be effective for inactivating pathogens in platelets and plasma, and is under development for application to whole blood. Because platelets and red blood cells do not contain a nucleus (i.e. they have no DNA to be damaged) the technique is well-suited for destroying nucleic acid containing pathogens (including viruses, bacteria, parasites, and white blood cells) in blood products.

Corneal ectasia is a progressive thinning of the cornea; the most common form of this condition is keratoconus. Collagen cross-linking is a non-surgical treatment intended to slow progression of corneal ectasia by strengthening corneal tissue. The standard protocol calls for application directly to the eye of a 0.1% riboflavin solution for 30 minutes followed by 30 minutes of ultraviolet-A irradiation with a wavelength of 370 nm and power of 3 mW/cm^2.

Side Effects

In humans, there is no evidence for riboflavin toxicity produced by excessive intakes, in part because it has lower water solubility than other B vitamins, because absorption becomes less efficient as doses increase, and because what excess is absorbed is excreted via the kidneys into urine. Even when 400 mg of riboflavin per day was given orally to subjects in one study for three months to investigate the efficacy of riboflavin in the prevention of migraine headache, no short-term side effects were reported. Although toxic doses can be administered by injection, any excess at nutritionally relevant doses is excreted in the urine, imparting a bright yellow color when in large quantities.

The Food and Nutrition Board of the U.S. Institute of Medicine sets Tolerable Upper Intake Levels (known as ULs) for vitamins and minerals when evidence is sufficient. In the case of riboflavin there is no UL, as there is no human data for adverse effects from high doses. The European Food Safety Authority reviewed the same safety question and also reached the conclusion that there was not sufficient evidence to set a UL for riboflavin.

Function

Riboflavin functions as a coenzyme, meaning that it is required for enzymes (proteins) to perform normal physiological actions. Specifically, the active forms of riboflavin flavin mononucleotide (FMN) and flavin adenine dinucleotide (FAD) function as cofactors for a variety of flavoproteine enzyme reactions:

- Flavoproteins of electron transport chain, including FMN in Complex I and FAD in Complex II
- FAD is required for the production of pyridoxic acid from pyridoxal (vitamin B_6) by pyridoxine 5'-phosphate oxidase
- The primary coenzyme form of vitamin B_6 (pyridoxal phosphate) is FMN dependent
- Oxidation of pyruvate, α-ketoglutarate, and branched-chain amino acids requires FAD in the shared E3 portion of their respective dehydrogenase complexes
- Fatty acyl CoA dehydrogenase requires FAD in fatty acid oxidation
- FAD is required to convert retinol (vitamin A) to retinoic acid via cytosolic retinal dehydrogenase
- Synthesis of an active form of folate (5-methyltetrahydrofolate) from 5,10-methylenetetrahydrofolate by Methylenetetrahydrofolate reductase is $FADH_2$ dependent
- FAD is required to convert tryptophan to niacin (vitamin B_3)
- Reduction of the oxidized form of glutathione (GSSG) to its reduced form (GSH) by Glutathione reductase is FAD dependent

Food Sources

Food and beverages that provide riboflavin without fortification are milk, cheese, eggs, leaf vegetables, liver, kidneys, legumes, mushrooms, and almonds.

The milling of cereals results in considerable loss (up to 60%) of vitamin B_2, so white flour is enriched in some countries such as US by addition of the vitamin. The enrichment of bread and ready-to-eat breakfast cereals contributes significantly to the dietary supply of vitamin B_2. Polished rice is not usually enriched, because the vitamin's yellow color would make the rice visually unacceptable to the major rice-consumption populations. However, most of the flavin content of whole brown rice is retained if the rice is steamed (parboiled) prior to milling. This process drives the flavins in the germ and aleurone layers into the endosperm. Free riboflavin is naturally present in foods along with protein-bound FMN and FAD. Bovine milk contains mainly free riboflavin, with a minor contribution from FMN and FAD. In whole milk, 14% of the flavins are bound noncovalently to specific proteins. Egg white and egg yolk contain specialized riboflavin-binding proteins, which are required for storage of free riboflavin in the egg for use by the developing embryo.

Riboflavin is added to baby foods, breakfast cereals, pastas and vitamin-enriched meal replacement products. It is difficult to incorporate riboflavin into liquid products because it has poor solubility in water, hence the requirement for riboflavin-5'-phosphate (E101a), a more soluble form of riboflavin. Riboflavin is also used as a food coloring and as such is designated in Europe as the E number E101.

Dietary Reference Intake

The Food and Nutrition Board of the U.S. Institute of Medicine updated Estimated Average Requirements (EARs) and Recommended Dietary Allowances (RDAs) in 1998. The current EARs for riboflavin for women and men ages 14 and up are 0.9 mg/day and 1.1 mg/day, respectively; the RDAs are 1.1 and 1.3 mg/day. RDAs are higher than EARs so as to identify amounts that will cover people with higher than average requirements. RDA for pregnancy equals 1.4 mg/day. RDA for lactation equals 1.6 mg/day. For infants up to 12 months the Adequate Intake (AI) is 0.3-0.4 mg/day and for children ages 1–13 years the RDA increases with age from 0.5 to 0.9 mg/day. Collectively the EARs, RDAs and ULs are referred to as Dietary Reference Intakes.

For U.S. food and dietary supplement labeling purposes the amount in a serving is expressed as a percent of Daily Value (%DV). For riboflavin labeling purposes 100% of the Daily Value was 1.7 mg, but as of May 2016 it has been revised to 1.3 mg. A table of the old and new adult Daily Values is provided at Reference Daily Intake. Food and supplement companies have until July 2018 to comply with the change.

Deficiency

Humans

Mild deficiencies can exceed 50% of the population in third world countries and in refugee situations. Deficiency is uncommon in the United States and in other countries that have wheat flour, bread, pasta, corn meal or rice enrichment regulations. In the U.S., starting in the 1940s, flour, corn meal and rice have been fortified with B vitamins as a means of restoring some of what is lost in milling, bleaching and other processing. For adults 20 and older, average intake from food and beverages is 1.8 mg/day for women and 2.5 mg/day for men. An estimated 23% consume a riboflavin-containing dietary supplement that provides on average 10 mg. The U.S. Department of Health and Human Services conducts National Health and Nutrition Examination Survey every two years and reports food results in a series of reports referred to as "What We Eat In America." From NHANES 2011–2012, the latest for which data has been reported, estimates are that 8% of women and 3% of men consume less than the RDA. When compared to the lower Estimated Average Requirements, fewer than 3% do not achieve the EAR level. However, anyone choosing a gluten-free or low gluten diet should as a precaution take a multi-vitamin/mineral dietary supplement which provides 100% DV for riboflavin and other B vitamins.

Riboflavin deficiency (also called ariboflavinosis) results in stomatitis including painful red tongue with sore throat, chapped and fissured lips (cheilosis), and inflammation of the corners of the mouth (angular stomatitis). There can be oily scaly skin rashes on the scrotum, vulva, philtrum of the lip, or the nasolabial folds. The eyes can become itchy, watery, bloodshot and sensitive to light. Due to interference with iron absorption, even mild to moderate riboflavin deficiency results in an anemia with normal cell size and normal hemoglobin content (i.e. normochromic normocytic anemia). This is distinct from anemia caused by deficiency of folic acid (B_9) or cyanocobalamin (B_{12}), which causes anemia with large blood cells (megaloblastic anemia). Deficiency of riboflavin during pregnancy can result in birth defects including congenital heart defects and limb deformities.

The stomatitis symptoms are similar to those seen in pellagra, which is caused by niacin (B_3) deficiency. Therefore, riboflavin deficiency is sometimes called "pellagra sine pellagra" (pellagra without pellagra), because it causes stomatitis but not widespread peripheral skin lesions characteristic of niacin deficiency.

Riboflavin has been noted to prolong recovery from malaria, despite preventing growth of plasmodium (the malaria parasite).

Other Animals

In other animals, riboflavin deficiency results in lack of growth, failure to thrive, and eventual death. Experimental riboflavin deficiency in dogs results in growth failure, weakness, ataxia, and inability to stand. The animals collapse, become comatose, and die. During the deficiency state, dermatitis develops together with hair loss. Other signs include corneal opacity, lenticular cataracts, hemorrhagic adrenals, fatty degeneration of the kidney and liver, and inflammation of the mucous membrane of the gastrointestinal tract. Post-mortem studies in rhesus monkeys fed a riboflavin-deficient diet revealed about one-third the normal amount of riboflavin was present in the liver, which is the main storage organ for riboflavin in mammals. Riboflavin deficiency in birds results in low egg hatch rates.

Diagnosis

Overt clinical signs are rarely seen among inhabitants of the developed countries. The assessment of Riboflavin status is essential for confirming cases with unspecific symptoms where deficiency is suspected.

- Glutathione reductase is a nicotinamide adenine dinucleotide phosphate (NADPH) and FAD-dependent enzyme, and the major flavoprotein in erythrocyte. The measurement of the activity coefficient of erythrocyte glutathione reductase (EGR) is the preferred method for assessing riboflavin status. It provides a measure of tissue saturation and long-term riboflavin status. In vitro enzyme activity in terms of activity coefficients (AC) is determined both with and without the addition of FAD to the medium. ACs represent a ratio of the enzyme's activity with

FAD to the enzyme's activity without FAD. An AC of 1.2 to 1.4, riboflavin status is considered low when FAD is added to stimulate enzyme activity. An AC > 1.4 suggests riboflavin deficiency. On the other hand, if FAD is added and AC is < 1.2, then riboflavin status is considered acceptable. Tillotson and Bashor reported that a decrease in the intakes of riboflavin was associated with increase in EGR AC. In the UK study of Norwich elderly, initial EGR AC values for both males and females were significantly correlated with those measured 2 years later, suggesting that EGR AC may be a reliable measure of long-term biochemical riboflavin status of individuals. These findings are consistent with earlier studies.

- Experimental balance studies indicate that urinary riboflavin excretion rates increase slowly with increasing intakes, until intake level approach 1.0 mg/d, when tissue saturation occurs. At higher intakes, the rate of excretion increases dramatically. Once intakes of 2.5 mg/d are reached, excretion becomes approximately equal to the rate of absorption (Horwitt et al., 1950) (18). At such high intake a significant proportion of the riboflavin intake is not absorbed. If urinary riboflavin excretion is <19 μg/g creatinine (without recent riboflavin intake) or < 40 μg per day are indicative of deficiency.

Causes

Riboflavin is continuously excreted in the urine of healthy individuals, making deficiency relatively common when dietary intake is insufficient. Riboflavin deficiency is usually found together with other nutrient deficiencies, particularly of other water-soluble vitamins. A deficiency of riboflavin can be primary - poor vitamin sources in one's daily diet - or secondary, which may be a result of conditions that affect absorption in the intestine, the body not being able to use the vitamin, or an increase in the excretion of the vitamin from the body. Subclinical deficiency has also been observed in women taking oral contraceptives, in the elderly, in people with eating disorders, chronic alcoholism and in diseases such as HIV, inflammatory bowel disease, diabetes and chronic heart disease. The Celiac Disease Foundation points out that a gluten-free diet may be low in riboflavin (and other nutrients) as enriched wheat flour and wheat foods (bread, pasta, cereals, etc.) is a major dietary contribution to total riboflavin intake. Phototherapy to treat jaundice in infants can cause increased degradation of riboflavin, leading to deficiency if not monitored closely.

Treatment

Treatment involves a diet which includes an adequate amount of riboflavin containing foods. Multi-vitamin and mineral dietary supplements often contain 100% of the Daily Value for riboflavin, and can be used by persons concerned about an inadequate diet. Over-the-counter dietary supplements are available in the United States with doses as high as 100 mg (5882% of Daily Value), but there is no evidence that these high doses have any additional benefit for healthy people.

Chemistry

As a chemical compound, riboflavin is a yellow-orange solid substance with poor solubility in water compared to other B vitamins. Visually, it imparts color to vitamin supplements (and bright yellow color to the urine of persons taking a lot of it).

Industrial uses

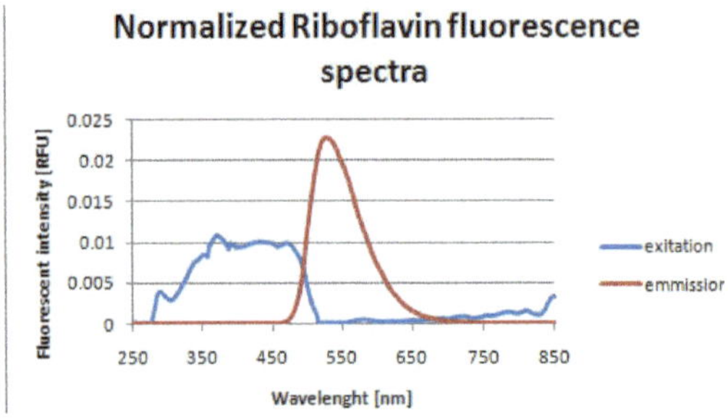

Fluorescent spectra of riboflavin

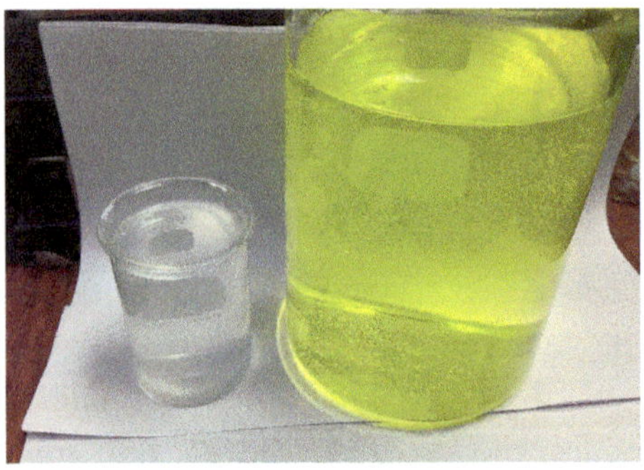

A solution of riboflavin in water (right) is yellow with chartreuse fluorescence under fluorescent room lighting. The beaker prepared at left holds a detergent in water, forming micelles that will show the passage of a visible laser beam.

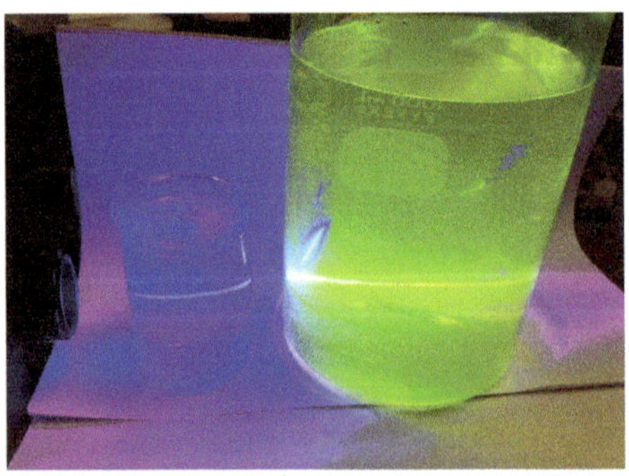

A 473 nm 200 mW blue laser beam is directed into the two beakers from the left. The detergent shows the path of the beam by blue scattered light. The light from the riboflavin solution is intense green fluorescence showing along the path of this laser beam.

Because riboflavin is fluorescent under UV light, dilute solutions (0.015-0.025% w/w) are often used to detect leaks or to demonstrate coverage in an industrial system such a chemical blend tank or bioreactor.

Industrial Synthesis

Various biotechnological processes have been developed for industrial scale riboflavin biosynthesis using different microorganisms, including filamentous fungi such as *Ashbya gossypii*, *Candida famata* and *Candida flaveri*, as well as the bacteria *Corynebacterium ammoniagenes* and *Bacillus subtilis*. The latter organism has been genetically modified to both increase the bacteria's production of riboflavin and to introduce an antibiotic (ampicillin) resistance marker, and is now successfully employed at a commercial scale to produce riboflavin for feed and food fortification purposes. The chemical company BASF has installed a plant in South Korea, which is specialized on riboflavin production using *Ashbya gossypii*. The concentrations of riboflavin in their modified strain are so high, that the mycelium has a reddish/brownish color and accumulates riboflavin crystals in the vacuoles, which will eventually burst the mycelium. Riboflavin is sometimes overproduced, possibly as a protective mechanism, by certain bacteria in the presence of high concentrations of hydrocarbons or aromatic compounds. One such organism is *Micrococcus luteus* (American Type Culture Collection strain number ATCC 49442), which develops a yellow color due to production of riboflavin while growing on pyridine, but not when grown on other substrates, such as succinic acid.

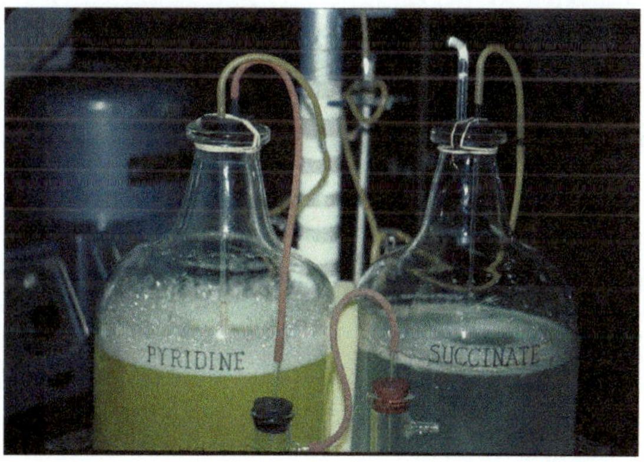

Large cultures of *Micrococcus luteus* growing on pyridine (left) and succinic acid (right). The yellow pigment being produced in the presence of pyridine is riboflavin.

History

Vitamin B was originally considered to have two components, a heat-labile vitamin B_1 and a heat-stable vitamin B_2. In the 1920s, vitamin B_2 was thought to be the factor necessary for preventing pellagra. In 1923, Paul Gyorgy in Heidelberg was investigating egg-white injury in rats; the curative factor for this condition was called vitamin H (which is now called biotin or vitamin B7). Since both pellagra and vitamin H deficiency were associated with dermatitis, Gyorgy decided to test the effect of vitamin B_2 on vitamin H deficiency in rats. He enlisted the service of Wagner-Jauregg in Kuhn's laboratory. In 1933, Kuhn, Gyorgy, and Wagner found that thiamin-free extracts of yeast, liver, or rice bran prevented the growth failure of rats fed a thiamin-supplemented diet.

Further, the researchers noted that a yellow-green fluorescence in each extract promoted rat growth, and that the intensity of fluorescence was proportional to the effect on growth. This observation enabled them to develop a rapid chemical and bioassay to isolate the factor from egg white in 1933, they called it Ovoflavin. The same group then isolated the same preparation (a growth-promoting compound with yellow-green fluorescence) from whey using the same procedure (lactoflavin). In 1934 Kuhn's group identified the structure of so-called flavin and synthesized vitamin B_2.

Name

The name "riboflavin" (often abbreviated to Rbf or RBF) comes from "ribose" (the sugar whose reduced form, ribitol, forms part of its structure) and "flavin", the ring-moiety which imparts the yellow color to the oxidized molecule (from Latin *flavus*, "yellow"). The reduced form, which occurs in metabolism along with the oxidized form, is colorless.

Vitamin B_6

Vitamin B_6 refers to a group of chemically similar compounds which can be interconverted in biological systems. Vitamin B_6 is part of the vitamin B group of essential nutrients. Its active form, pyridoxal 5′-phosphate, serves as a coenzyme in some 100 enzyme reactions in amino acid, glucose, and lipid metabolism.

Forms

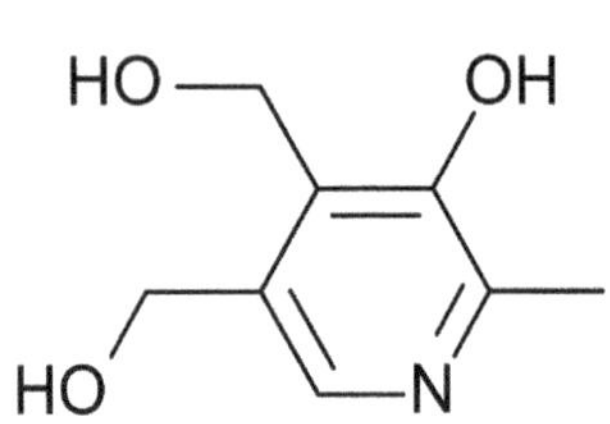

Pyridoxine

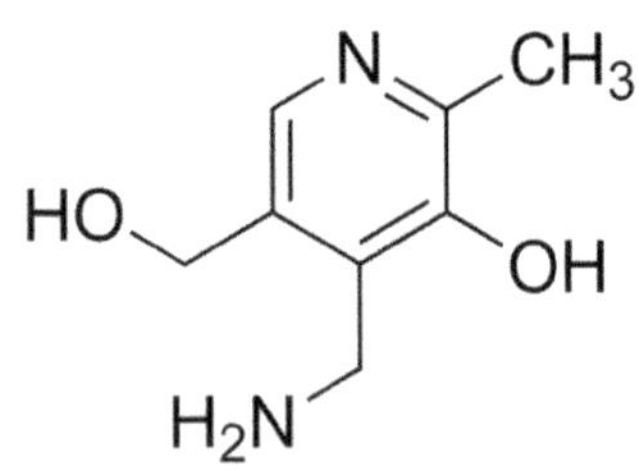

Pyridoxamine

Several forms (vitamers) of vitamin B_6 are known:

- Pyridoxine (PN), the form most commonly given as vitamin B_6 supplement
- Pyridoxine 5′-phosphate (P5P)
- Pyridoxal (PL)
- Pyridoxal 5′-phosphate (PLP), the metabolically active form (sold as P-5-P vitamin supplement)
- Pyridoxamine (PM)

- Pyridoxamine 5′-phosphate (PMP)
- 4-Pyridoxic acid (PA), the catabolite which is excreted in urine
- Pyritinol, a semi-synthetic derivative of pyridoxine, where two pyridoxine moieties are bound by a disulfide bridge.

All forms except pyridoxic acid and pyritinol can be interconverted. Absorbed pyridoxamine is converted to PMP by pyridoxal kinase, which is further converted to PLP by pyridoxamine-phosphate transaminase or pyridoxine 5′-phosphate oxidase which also catalyzes the conversion of PNP to PLP. Pyridoxine 5′-phosphate oxidase is dependent on flavin mononucleotide (FMN) as a cofactor which is produced from riboflavin (vitamin B_2) i.e. in this biochemical pathway, dietary vitamin B_6 cannot be used without vitamin B_2.

Functions

PLP, the metabolically active form of vitamin B_6, is involved in many aspects of macronutrient metabolism, neurotransmitter synthesis, histamine synthesis, hemoglobin synthesis and function, and gene expression. PLP generally serves as a coenzyme (cofactor) for many reactions including decarboxylation, transamination, racemization, elimination, replacement, and beta-group interconversion. The liver is the site for vitamin B_6 metabolism.

Amino Acid Metabolism

1. PLP is a cofactor in the biosynthesis of five important neurotransmitters: serotonin, dopamine, epinephrine, norepinephrine, and gamma-aminobutyric acid (GABA). PLP is also involved in the synthesis of histamine.
2. Transaminases break down amino acids with PLP as a cofactor. The proper activity of these enzymes is crucial for the process of moving amine groups from one amino acid to another.
3. Serine racemase which synthesizes the neuromodulator d-serine from its eiantiomer is a PLP-dependent enzyme.
4. PLP is a coenzyme needed for the proper function of the enzymes cystathionine synthase and cystathionase. These enzymes catalyze reactions in the catabolism of methionine. Part of this pathway (the reaction catalyzed by cystathionase) also produces cysteine.
5. Selenomethionine is the primary dietary form of selenium. PLP is needed as a cofactor for the enzymes that allow selenium to be used from the dietary form. PLP also plays a cofactor role in releasing selenium from selenohomocysteine to produce hydrogen selenide, which can then be used to incorporate selenium into selenoproteins.

6. PLP is required for the conversion of tryptophan to niacin, so low vitamin B_6 status impairs this conversion.

Glucose Metabolism

PLP is a required coenzyme of glycogen phosphorylase, the enzyme necessary for glycogenolysis to occur. PLP can catalyze transamination reactions that are essential for providing amino acids as a substrate for gluconeogenesis.

Lipid Metabolism

PLP is an essential component of enzymes that facilitate the biosynthesis of sphingolipids. Particularly, the synthesis of ceramide requires PLP. In this reaction, serine is decarboxylated and combined with palmitoyl-CoA to form sphinganine, which is combined with a fatty acyl-CoA to form dihydroceramide. Dihydroceramide is then further desaturated to form ceramide. In addition, the breakdown of sphingolipids is also dependent on vitamin B_6 because sphingosine-1-phosphate lyase, the enzyme responsible for breaking down sphingosine-1-phosphate, is also PLP-dependent.

Hemoglobin Synthesis and Function

PLP aids in the synthesis of hemoglobin, by serving as a coenzyme for the enzyme ALA synthase. It also binds to two sites on hemoglobin to enhance the oxygen binding of hemoglobin.

Gene Expression

PLP has been implicated in increasing or decreasing the expression of certain genes. Increased intracellular levels of the vitamin lead to a decrease in the transcription of glucocorticoids. Also, vitamin B_6 deficiency leads to the increased gene expression of albumin mRNA. Also, PLP influences expression of glycoprotein IIb by interacting with various transcription factors. The result is inhibition of platelet aggregation.

Nutrition

Food Sources

Vitamin B_6 is widely distributed in foods in both its free and bound forms. Cooking, storage, and processing losses of vitamin B_6 vary and in some foods may be more than 50%, depending on the form of vitamin present in the food. Plant foods lose the least during processing, as they contain mostly pyridoxine, which is far more stable than the pyridoxal or pyridoxamine found in animal foods. For example, milk can lose 30–70% of its vitamin B_6 content when dried. Vitamin B_6 is found in the germ and aleurone layer of grains, and milling results in the reduction of this vitamin in white flour. The heating that occurs before most freezing and canning processes are other methods that may result in the loss of vitamin B_6 in foods.

Foods that contain large amounts of vitamin B_6 include

- fortified breakfast cereals
- pork
- turkey
- beef
- bananas
- chickpeas
- potatoes
- pistachios

Dietary Reference Intake

The Food and Nutrition Board (FNB) of the U.S. Institute of Medicine updated Estimated Average Requirements (EARs) and Recommended Dietary Allowances (RDAs) for vitamin B_6 in 1998. The current EARs for vitamin B_6 for women and men ages 14 and up increase with age from 1.0 to 1.3 mg/day and from 1.1 to 1.4 mg/day, respectively; the RDAs increase with age from 1.2 to 1.5 and from 1.3 to 1.7 mg/day, respectively. RDAs are higher than EARs so as to identify amounts that will cover people with higher than average requirements. RDA for pregnancy equals 1.9 mg/day. RDA for lactation equals 2.0 mg/day. For infants up to 12 months the Adequate Intake (AI) is 0.1–0.3 mg/day. and for children ages 1–13 years the RDA increases with age from 0.5 to 1.0 mg/day. As for safety, the FNB sets Tolerable Upper Intake Levels (known as ULs) for vitamins and minerals when evidence is sufficient. In the case of vitamin B_6 the UL is set at 100 mg/day. The European Food Safety Authority reviewed the same safety question and set its UL at 25 mg/day. Safety issues are presented at length in the Toxicity section. Collectively the EARs, RDAs, AIs and ULs are referred to as Dietary Reference Intakes.

For U.S. food and dietary supplement labeling purposes the amount in a serving is expressed as a percent of daily value (%DV). For vitamin B_6 labeling purposes 100% of the Daily Value was 2.0 mg, but as of May 2016 it has been revised to 1.7 mg. A table of the old and new adult Daily Values is provided at Reference Daily Intake. Food and supplement companies have until July 28, 2018 to comply with the change.

Absorption and Excretion

Vitamin B_6 is absorbed in the jejunum and ileum by passive diffusion. With the capacity for absorption being so great, animals are able to absorb quantities much greater than necessary for physiological demands. The absorption of pyridoxal phosphate and pyridoxamine phosphate involves their dephosphorylation catalyzed by a membrane-bound alkaline phosphatase. Those products and nonphosphorylated forms in the digestive tract are absorbed by diffusion, which is driven by trapping of the vitamin as 5′-phosphates through the action of phosphorylation (by a pyridoxal kinase) in the jejunal mucosa. The trapped pyridoxine and pyridoxamine are oxidized to pyridoxal phosphate in the tissue.

The products of vitamin B_6 metabolism are excreted in the urine, the major product of which is 4-pyridoxic acid. An estimated 40–60% of ingested vitamin B_6 is oxidized to 4-pyridoxic acid. Several studies have shown that 4-pyridoxic acid is undetectable in the urine of vitamin B_6-deficient subjects, making it a useful clinical marker to assess the vitamin B_6 status of an individual. Other products of vitamin B_6 metabolism excreted in the urine when high doses of the vitamin have been given include pyridoxal, pyridoxamine, and pyridoxine and their phosphates. A small amount of vitamin B_6 is also excreted in the feces.

Deficiency

Signs and Symptoms

The classic clinical syndrome for vitamin B_6 deficiency is a seborrhoeic dermatitis-like eruption, atrophic glossitis with ulceration, angular cheilitis, conjunctivitis, intertrigo, and neurologic symptoms of somnolence, confusion, and neuropathy (due to impaired sphingosine synthesis) and sideroblastic anemia (due to impaired heme synthesis).

Less severe cases present with metabolic disease associated with insufficient activities of the coenzyme PLP. The most prominent of the lesions is due to impaired tryptophan–niacin conversion. This can be detected based on urinary excretion of xanthurenic acid after an oral tryptophan load. Vitamin B_6 deficiency can also result in impaired trans-sulfuration of methionine to cysteine. The PLP-dependent transaminases and glycogen phosphorylase provide the vitamin with its role in gluconeogenesis, so deprivation of vitamin B_6 results in impaired glucose tolerance.

Diagnosis

The assessment of vitamin B_6 status is essential, as the clinical signs and symptoms in less severe cases are not specific. The three biochemical tests most widely used are the activation coefficient for the erythrocyte enzyme aspartate aminotransferase, plasma PLP concentrations, and the urinary excretion of vitamin B_6 degradation products, specifically urinary PA. Of these, plasma PLP is probably the best single measure, because it reflects tissue stores. Plasma PLP less than 10 nmol/l is indicative of vitamin B_6 deficiency. A PLP concentration greater than 20 nmol/l has been chosen as a level of adequacy for establishing Estimated Average Requirements and Recommended Daily Allowances in the USA. Urinary PA is also an indicator of vitamin B_6 deficiency; levels of less than 3.0 mmol/day is suggestive of vitamin B_6 deficiency.

The classic syndrome for vitamin B_6 deficiency is rare, even in developing countries. A handful of cases were seen between 1952 and 1953, particularly in the United States, and occurred in a small percentage of infants who were fed a formula lacking in pyridoxine.

Causes

A deficiency of vitamin B_6 alone is relatively uncommon and often occurs in association with other vitamins of the B complex. The elderly and alcoholics have an increased risk of vitamin B_6 deficiency, as well as other micronutrient deficiencies. Evidence exists for decreased levels of vitamin B_6 in women with type 1 diabetes and in patients with systemic inflammation, liver disease, rheumatoid arthritis, and those infected with HIV. Use of oral contraceptives and treatment with certain anticonvulsants, isoniazid, cycloserine, penicillamine, and hydrocortisone negatively impact vitamin B_6 status. Hemodialysis reduces vitamin B_6 plasma levels.

There are indications that B_6 deficiency can be influenced by theophylline in medication or malnutrition.

Treatment

Treatment of vitamin B_6 deficiency lies with replacement, usually in the form of pyridoxine hydrochloride, orally, as a nasal spray, or for injection when in its solution form.

Side Effects

Adverse effects have been documented from vitamin B_6 supplements, but never from food sources. Toxicologic animal studies identify specific destruction of the dorsal root ganglia which is documented in human cases of overdose of pyridoxine. Although it is a water-soluble vitamin and is excreted in the urine, doses of pyridoxine in excess of the RDI over long periods of time result in painful and ultimately irreversible neurological problems.

The primary symptoms are pain and numbness of the extremities. In severe cases, motor neuropathy may occur with "slowing of motor conduction velocities, prolonged F wave latencies, and prolonged sensory latencies in both lower extremities", causing difficulty in walking. Sensory neuropathy typically develops at doses of pyridoxine in excess of 1,000 mg per day, but adverse effects can occur with much less, so doses over 200 mg are not considered safe. Symptoms among women taking lower doses have been reported. Two reported cases of neuropathy with pyridoxine treatment of 24 and 40 mg/day may have been coincidental.

Existing authorizations and valuations vary considerably worldwide. In 1993, the European Community Scientific Committee on Food defined intakes of 50 mg of vitamin B_6 per day as harmful and established a tolerable upper intake level of 25 mg/day for adults in 2000. The Expert Group on Vitamins and Minerals of the Food Standard Agency UK (UK EVM) derived a safe upper level (SUL) of 10 mg/day for a 60 kg adult in 2003. The tolerable upper limit has been set by the US FDA at 100 mg/day in 2000.

The nutrient reference values in Australia and New Zealand recommend an upper limit of 50 mg a day in adults. "The same figure was set for pregnancy and lactation as there is no evidence of teratogenicity at this level. The UL was set based on metabolic body size and growth considerations for all other ages and life stages except infancy. It was not possible to set a UL for infants, so intake is recommended in the form of food, milk or formula." "The ULs were set using results of studies involving long-term oral administration of pyridoxine at doses of less than 1 g/day. A no-observed-adverse-effect level (NOAEL) of 200 mg/day was identified from the studies of Bernstein & Lobitz (1988) and Del Tredici *et al* (1985). These studies involved subjects who had generally been on the supplements for five to six months or less. The study of Dalton and Dalton (1987), however, suggested the symptoms might take substantially longer than this to appear. In this latter retrospective survey, subjects who reported symptoms had been on supplements for 2.9 years, on average. Those reporting no symptoms had taken supplements for 1.9 years."

Because no placebo-controlled studies show therapeutic benefits of high doses of pyridoxine, and the well-documented occurrence of significant toxic effects, little reason exists to exceed the RDI using supplements unless under medical supervision (e.g. in treatment of primary hyperoxaluria).

History

In 1934, the Hungarian physician Paul György discovered a substance that was able to cure a skin disease in rats (dermititis acrodynia). He named this substance vitamin B_6. In 1938, Samuel Lepkovsky isolated vitamin B_6 from rice bran. Harris and Folkers in 1939 determined the structure of pyridoxine, and, in 1945, Snell was able to show the two forms of vitamin B_6, pyridoxal and pyridoxamine. Vitamin B_6 was named pyridoxine to indicate its structural homology to pyridine.

Biotin Deficiency

Biotin deficiency is a rare nutritional disorder which can become serious, even fatal, if allowed to progress untreated. It can occur in people of any age, ancestry, or gender. Biotin is part of the B vitamin family. Biotin deficiency rarely occurs among healthy people because the daily requirement of biotin is low, many foods provide adequate amounts of it, intestinal bacteria synthesize small amounts of it, and the body effectively scavenges and recycles it from bodily waste. However, deficiencies can be caused by consuming raw egg whites over a period of months to years. Egg whites contain high levels of avidin, a protein that binds biotin strongly. When cooked, avidin is partially denatured and binding to biotin is reduced. However one study showed that 30-40% of the avidin activity was still present in the white after frying or boiling. But cooked egg whites are safer to consume. Genetic disorders such as Biotinidase deficiency, Multiple carboxylase deficiency, and Holocarboxylase synthetase deficiency can also lead to inborn or late-onset forms of biotin deficiency. In all cases – dietary, genetic, or otherwise – supplementation with biotin is the primary method of treatment.

Biochemistry

Biotin is a coenzyme for five carboxylases in the human body (propionyl-CoA carboxylase, methylcrotonyl-CoA carboxylase, pyruvate carboxylase, and 2 forms of acetyl-CoA carboxylase.) Therefore, biotin is essential for amino acid catabolism, gluconeogenesis, and fatty acid metabolism. Biotin is also necessary for gene stability because it is covalently attached to histones. Biotinylated histones play a role in repression of transposable elements and some genes. Normally, the amount of biotin in the body is regulated by dietary intake, biotin transporters (monocarboxylate transporter 1 and sodium-dependent multivitamin transporter), peptidyl hydrolase biotinidase (BTD), and the protein ligase holocarboxylase synthetase. When any of these regulatory factors are inhibited, biotin deficiency could occur.

Signs and Symptoms

- Rashes including red, patchy ones near the mouth (erythematous periorofacial macular rash)
- Fine and brittle hair
- Hair loss or total baldness (alopecia)
- Anemia
- Birth Defects (still being studied)
- Seborrheic dermatitis
- Fungal infections

Psychological

- Hallucinations
- Lethargy
- Anorexia
- Mild depression, which may progress to profound fatigue and, eventually, to somnolence
- Generalized muscular pains (myalgias)
- Paresthesias

Causes

1. Total parenteral nutrition without biotin supplementation: Several cases of biotin deficiency in patients receiving prolonged total parenteral nutrition (TPN) therapy without added biotin have been reported. Therefore, all patients receiving TPN must also receive biotin at the recommended daily dose, especially if TPN therapy is expected to last more than 1 week. All hospital pharmacies currently include biotin in TPN preparations.

2. Protein deficiency: A shortage of proteins involved in biotin homeostasis can cause biotin deficiency. The main proteins involved in biotin homeostasis are HCS, BTD (biotinidase deficiency) and SMVT

3. Anticonvulsant therapy: Prolonged use of certain drugs (especially highly common prescription anti-seizure medications such as phenytoin, primidone, and carbamazepine), may lead to biotin deficiency; however, valproic acid therapy is less likely to cause this condition. Some anticonvulsants inhibit biotin transport across the intestinal mucosa. Evidence suggests that these anticonvulsants accelerate biotin catabolism, which means that it's necessary for people to take supplemental biotin, in addition to the usual minimum daily requirements, if they're treated with anticonvulsant medication(s) that have been linked to biotin deficiency.

4. Severe Malnourishment

5. Prolonged oral antibiotic therapy: Prolonged use of oral antibiotics has been associated with biotin deficiency. Alterations in the intestinal flora caused by the prolonged administration of antibiotics are presumed to be the basis for biotin deficiency.

6. Genetic mutation: Mikati et al. (2006) reported a case of partial biotinidase deficiency (plasma biotinidase level of 1.3 nm/min/mL) in a 7-month-old boy. The boy presented with perinatal distress followed by developmental delay, hypotonia, seizures, and infantile spasms without alopecia or dermatitis. The child's neurologic symptoms abated following biotin supplementation and antiepileptic drug therapy. DNA mutational analysis revealed that the child was homozygous for a novel E64K mutation and that his mother and father were heterozygous for the novel E64K mutation.

7. Pregnancy

Potential Causes

1. Smoking: Recent studies suggest that smoking can lead to marginal biotin deficiency because it speeds up biotin catabolism (especially in women).

2. Excessive alcohol consumption

3. Excessive consumption of antidiuretics or inadequate levels of antidiuretic hormone
4. Intestinal malabsorption caused by short bowel syndrome
5. Ketogenic Diet

Diagnosis

The most reliable and commonly used methods for determining biotin status in the body are:

- excretion of 3-hydroxyisovaleric acid and biotin in urine
- activity of propionyl-CoA carboxylase in lymphocytes

Treatment

In the United States biotin supplements are readily available without a prescription in amounts ranging from 1,000 to 10,000 micrograms (30 micrograms is identified as Adequate Intake).

Epidemiology

Since biotin is in many foods at low concentrations, deficiency is rare except in locations where malnourishment is very common. Pregnancy, however, alters biotin catabolism and despite a regular biotin intake, half of the pregnant women in the U.S. are marginally biotin deficient.

Folate Deficiency

Folate deficiency is a low level of folic acid and derivatives in the body. Also known as vitamin B9, folate is involved in adenosine, guanine, and thymidine synthesis (part of DNA synthesis). Signs of folate deficiency are often subtle. Anemia is a late finding in folate deficiency and folate deficiency anemia is the term given for this medical condition. It is characterized by the appearance of large-sized, abnormal red blood cells (megaloblasts), which form when there are inadequate stores of folic acid within the body.

Signs and symptoms

Loss of appetite and weight loss can occur. Additional signs are weakness, sore tongue, headaches, heart palpitations, irritability, and behavioral disorders. In adults, anemia (macrocytic, megaloblastic anemia) can be a sign of advanced folate deficiency.

In infants and children, folate deficiency can slow growth rate. Women with folate deficiency who become pregnant are more likely to give birth to low birth weight premature infants, and infants with neural tube defects.

Causes

A deficiency of folate can occur when the body's need for folate is increased, when dietary intake of folate is inadequate, or when the body excretes (or loses) more folate than usual. Medications that interfere with the body's ability to use folate may also increase the need for this vitamin. Some research indicates that exposure to ultraviolet light, including the use of tanning beds, can lead to a folate deficiency. The deficiency is more common in pregnant women, infants, children, and adolescents. May also be due to poor diet or a consequence of alcoholism.

Additionally, a defect in homocysteine methyltransferase or a deficiency of B-12 may lead to a so-called "methyl-trap" of tetrahydrofolate (THF), in which THF is converted to a reservoir of methyl-THF which thereafter has no way of being metabolized, and serves as a sink of THF that causes a subsequent deficiency in folate. Thus, a deficiency in B-12 can generate a large pool of methyl-THF that is unable to undergo reactions and will mimic folate deficiency.

Folate (pteroylmonoglutamate) is absorbed throughout the small intestine, though mainly in the Jejunum, binding to specific receptor proteins. Diffuse inflammatory or degenerative diseases of the small intestine, such as Crohn's disease, coeliac disease, chronic enteritis or entero-enteric fistulae, may reduce the activity of pteroyl polyglutamase (PPGH), a specific hydrolase required for folate absorption, and thereby leading to folate deficiency.

Situational

Some situations that increase the need for folate include the following:

- hemorrhage
- kidney dialysis
- liver disease
- malabsorption, including celiac disease and fructose malabsorption
- pregnancy and lactation (breastfeeding)
- tobacco smoking
- alcohol consumption

Medication

Medications can interfere with folate utilization, including:

- anticonvulsant medications (such as phenytoin, primidone, carbamazepine or valproate)

- metformin (sometimes prescribed to control blood sugar in type 2 diabetes)
- methotrexate, an anti-cancer drug also used to control inflammation associated with Crohn's disease, ulcerative colitis and rheumatoid arthritis.
- sulfasalazine (used to control inflammation associated with Crohn's disease, ulcerative colitis and rheumatoid arthritis)
- triamterene (a diuretic)
- birth control pills

When methotrexate is prescribed, folic acid supplements are sometimes given with the methotrexate. The therapeutic effects of methotrexate are due to its inhibition of dihydrofolate reductase and thereby reduce the rate *de novo* purine and pyrimidine synthesis and cell division. Methotrexate inhibits cell division and is particularly toxic to fast dividing cells, such as rapidly dividing cancer cells and the progenitor cells of the immune system. Folate supplementation is beneficial in patients being treated with long-term, low-dose methotrexate for inflammatory conditions, such as rheumatoid arthritis (RA) or psoriasis, to avoid macrocytic anemia caused by folate deficiency. Folate is often also supplemented before some high dose chemotherapy treatments in an effort to protect healthy tissue. However, it may be counterproductive to take a folic acid supplement with methotrexate in cancer treatment.

Prevention and Treatment

Folate is found in leafy green vegetables. Multi-vitamins also tend to include Folate as well as many other B vitamins. B vitamins, such as Folate, are water-soluble and excess is excreted in the urine.

When cooking, use of steaming or of a food steamer can help keep more folate content in the cooked foods, thus helping to prevent folate deficiency.

Folate deficiency during human pregnancy has been associated with an increased risk of infant neural tube defects. Such deficiency during the first four weeks of gestation can result in structural and developmental problems. NIH guidelines recommend oral B vitamin supplements to decrease these risks near the time of conception and during the first month of pregnancy.

Research

Folate deficiency during gestation or infancy due to development by the fetus or infant of autoantibodies to the folate receptor might result in various developmental disorders including autism spectrum disorders.

Studies suggest that insufficient folate and vitamin B_{12} status may contribute to major depressive disorder and that supplementation might be useful in this condition. The role of vitamin B_{12} and folate in depression is due to their role in transmethylation reactions, which are crucial for the formation of neurotransmitters (e.g. serotonin, epinephrine, nicotinamides, purines, phospholipids). The proposed mechanism, is that low levels of folate or vitamin B_{12} can disrupt transmethylation reaction, leading to an accumulation of homocysteine (hyperhomocisteinemia) and to impaired metabolism of neurotransmitters (especially the hydroxylation of dopamine and serotonin from tyrosine and tryptophan), phospholipids, myelin, and receptors. High homocysteine levels in the blood can lead to vascular injuries by oxidative mechanisms which can contribute to cerebral dysfunction. All of these can lead to the development of various disorders, including depression.

Vitamin B_{12} Deficiency

Vitamin B_{12} deficiency is the medical condition of low blood levels of vitamin B_{12}. A wide variety of signs and symptoms may occur including a decreased ability to think and behavioural and emotional changes such as depression, irritability, and psychosis. Abnormal sensations, changes in reflexes, and poor muscle function can also occur as may inflammation of the tongue, decreased taste, low red blood cells, reduced heart function, and decreased fertility. In young children symptoms include poor growth, poor development, and difficulties with movement. Without early treatment some of the changes may be permanent.

Common causes include poor absorption from the stomach or intestines, decreased intake, and increased requirements. Decreased absorption may be due to pernicious anemia, surgical removal of the stomach, chronic inflammation of the pancreas, intestinal parasites, certain medications, and some genetic disorders. Decreased intake may occur in those who eat a vegan diet or are malnourished. Increased requirements occur in HIV/AIDS and in those with rapid red blood cell breakdown. Diagnosis is typically based on vitamin B_{12} blood levels below 120–180 picomol/L (170–250 pg/mL) in adults. Elevated methylmalonic acid levels (values >0.4 micromol/L) may also indicate a deficiency. A type of low red blood cells known as megaloblastic anemia is often but not always present.

Supplementation is recommended to prevent deficiency in vegetarians who are pregnant. Once identified it is easily treated with supplementation by mouth or injection. There are no concerns from excess vitamin B_{12} among those who are otherwise healthy. Some cases may also be helped by treating the underlying cause. Other cases may require ongoing supplementation as the underlying cause is not curable. Vitamin B_{12} deficiency is common. It is estimated to occur in about 6% of those under the age of 60 and 20% of those over the age of 60. Rates may be as high as 80% in parts of Africa and Asia.

Signs and Symptoms

Vitamin B_{12} deficiency can lead to anemia and neurologic dysfunction. A mild deficiency may not cause any discernible symptoms, but as the deficiency becomes more significant, symptoms of anemia may result, such as weakness, fatigue, light-headedness, rapid heartbeat, rapid breathing and pale color to the skin. It may also cause easy bruising or bleeding, including bleeding gums. GI side effects including sore tongue, stomach upset, weight loss, and diarrhea or constipation. If the deficiency is not corrected, nerve cell damage can result. If this happens, vitamin B_{12} deficiency may result in tingling or numbness to the fingers and toes, difficulty walking, mood changes, depression, memory loss, disorientation and, in severe cases, dementia.

The main syndrome of vitamin B_{12} deficiency is pernicious anemia. It is characterized by a triad of symptoms:

1. Anemia with bone marrow promegaloblastosis (megaloblastic anemia). This is due to the inhibition of DNA synthesis (specifically purines and thymidine)
2. Gastrointestinal symptoms: alteration in bowel motility, such as mild diarrhea or constipation, and loss of bladder or bowel control. These are thought to be due to defective DNA synthesis inhibiting replication in a site with a high turnover of cells. This may also be due to the autoimmune attack on the parietal cells of the stomach in pernicious anemia. There is an association with GAVE syndrome (commonly called watermelon stomach) and pernicious anemia.
3. Neurological symptoms: Sensory or motor deficiencies (absent reflexes, diminished vibration or soft touch sensation), subacute combined degeneration of spinal cord, seizures, or even symptoms of dementia and or other psychiatric symptoms may be present. The presence of peripheral sensory-motor symptoms or subacute combined degeneration of spinal cord strongly suggests the presence of a B_{12} deficiency instead of folate deficiency. Methylmalonic acid, if not properly handled by B_{12}, remains in the myelin sheath, causing fragility. Dementia and depression have been associated with this deficiency as well, possibly from the under-production of methionine because of the inability to convert homocysteine into this product. Methionine is a necessary cofactor in the production of several neurotransmitters.

Each of those symptoms can occur either alone or along with others. The neurological complex, defined as *myelosis funicularis*, consists of the following symptoms:

1. Impaired perception of deep touch, pressure and vibration, loss of sense of touch, very annoying and persistent paresthesias
2. Ataxia of dorsal chord type
3. Decrease or loss of deep muscle-tendon reflexes
4. Pathological reflexes — Babinski, Rossolimo and others, also severe paresis

Vitamin B_{12} deficiency can cause severe and irreversible damage, especially to the brain and nervous system. These symptoms of neuronal damage may not reverse after correction of hematological abnormalities, and the chance of complete reversal decreases with the length of time the neurological symptoms have been present.

Tinnitus may be associated with vitamin B_{12} deficiency.

Psychological

Vitamin B_{12} deficiency can also cause symptoms of mania and psychosis, fatigue, memory impairment, irritability, depression, ataxia, and personality changes. In infants symptoms include irritability, failure to thrive, apathy, anorexia, and developmental regression.

Causes

- Inadequate dietary intake of vitamin B_{12}. Vitamin B_{12} occurs in animal products (eggs, meat, milk) and recent research indicates it may also occur in some algae, such as *Chlorella* and Susabi-nori (*Porphyra yezoensis*). B_{12} isolated from bacterial cultures is also added to many fortified foods, and available as a dietary supplement. Vegans, and also vegetarians but to a lesser degree, may be at risk for B_{12} deficiency due to inadequate dietary intake of B_{12}, if they do not supplement. However, B_{12} deficiency can occur even in people who consume meat, poultry, and fish. Children are at a higher risk for B_{12} deficiency due to inadequate dietary intake, as they have fewer vitamin stores and a relatively larger vitamin need per calorie of food intake.

- Selective impaired absorption of vitamin B_{12} due to intrinsic factor deficiency. This may be caused by the loss of gastric parietal cells in chronic atrophic gastritis (in which case, the resulting megaloblastic anemia takes the name of "pernicious anemia"), or may result from wide surgical resection of stomach (for any reason), or from rare hereditary causes of impaired synthesis of intrinsic factor.

- Impaired absorption of vitamin B_{12} in the setting of a more generalized malabsorption or maldigestion syndrome. This includes any form of structural damage or wide surgical resection of the terminal ileum (the principal site of vitamin B_{12} absorption).

- Forms of achlorhydria (including that artificially induced by drugs such as proton pump inhibitors and histamine 2 receptor antagonists) can cause B_{12} malabsorption from foods, since acid is needed to split B_{12} from food proteins and salivary binding proteins. This process is thought to be the most common cause of low B_{12} in the elderly, who often have some degree of achlorhydria without being formally low in intrinsic factor. This process does not affect absorption of small amounts of B_{12} in supplements such as multivitamins, since it is not bound to proteins, as is the B_{12} in foods.

- Surgical removal of the small bowel (for example in Crohn's disease) such that the patient presents with short bowel syndrome and is unable to absorb vitamin B_{12}. This can be treated with regular injections of vitamin B_{12}.
- Long-term use of ranitidine hydrochloride may contribute to deficiency of vitamin B_{12}.
- Untreated celiac disease may also cause impaired absorption of this vitamin, probably due to damage to the small bowel mucosa. In some people, vitamin B12 deficiency may persist despite treatment with a gluten-free diet and require supplementation.
- Some bariatric surgical procedures, especially those that involve removal of part of the stomach, such as Roux-en-Y gastric bypass surgery. (Procedures such as the adjustable gastric band type do not appear to affect B_{12} metabolism significantly).
- Bacterial overgrowth in parts of the small bowel are thought to be able to absorb B_{12}. An example occurs in so-called blind loop syndrome.
- The diabetes medication metformin may interfere with B_{12} dietary absorption.
- Hereditary causes such as severe MTHFR deficiency, homocystinuria, and transcobalamin deficiency.
- Malnutrition of alcoholism.
- Nitrous oxide abuse.
- Infection with the Diphyllobothrium latum tapeworm

Mechanism

The total amount of vitamin B_{12} stored in the body is between two and five milligrams in adults. Approximately 50% is stored in the liver, but approximately 0.1% is lost each day, due to secretions into the gut—not all of the vitamin in the gut is reabsorbed. While bile is the main vehicle for B_{12} excretion, most of the B_{12} secreted in bile is recycled via enterohepatic circulation. Due to the extreme efficiency of this mechanism, the liver can store three to five years worth of vitamin B_{12} under normal conditions and functioning. However, the rate at which B_{12} levels may change when dietary intake is low depends on the balance between several variables.

Metabolic

Vitamin B_{12} deficiency causes particular changes to the metabolism of 2 clinically relevant substances in humans:

1. Homocysteine (homocysteine to methionine, catalysed by methionine synthase) leading to hyperhomocysteinemia may lead to varicose veins

2. Methylmalonic acid (methylmalonyl-CoA to succinyl-CoA, of which methylmalonyl-CoA is made from methylmalonic acid in a preceding reaction)

Methionine is activated to *S*-adenosyl methionine, which aids in purine and thymidine synthesis, myelin production, protein/neurotransmitters/fatty acid/phospholipid production and DNA methylation. 5-Methyl tetrahydrofolate provides a methyl group, which is released to the reaction with homocysteine, resulting in methionine. This reaction requires cobalamin as a cofactor. The creation of 5-methyl tetrahydrofolate is an irreversible reaction. If B_{12} is absent, the forward reaction of homocysteine to methionine does not occur, and the replenishment of tetrahydrofolate stops.

Because B_{12} and folate are involved in the metabolism of homocysteine, hyperhomocysteinuria is a non-specific marker of deficiency. Methylmalonic acid is used as a more specific test of B_{12} deficiency.

Pathomorphology

A spongiform state of neural tissue along with edema of fibers and deficiency of tissue. The myelin decays, along with axial fiber. In later phases, fibric sclerosis of nervous tissues occurs. Those changes apply to dorsal parts of the spinal cord and to pyramidal tracts in lateral cords. The pathophysiologic state of the spinal cord is called subacute combined degeneration of spinal cord.

In the brain itself, changes are less severe: They occur as small sources of nervous fibers decay and accumulation of astrocytes, usually subcortically located, and also round hemorrhages with a torus of glial cells. Pathological changes can be noticed as well in the posterior roots of the cord and, to lesser extent, in peripheral nerves. Abnormalities might be observed in MRI.

Diagnosis

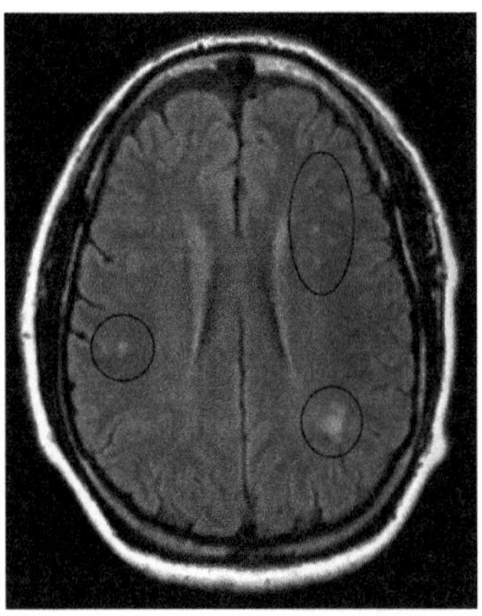

MRI image of the brain in an axial view showing the "precontrast FLAIR image". Note the abnormal lesions (circled) in the per ventricular area suggesting white matter pathology in someone with vitamin B12 deficiency.

Serum B_{12} levels are often low in B_{12} deficiency, but if other features of B_{12} deficiency are present with normal B_{12} then further investigation is warranted. One possible explanation for normal B_{12} levels in B_{12} deficiency is antibody interference in people with high titres of intrinsic factor antibody. Some researchers propose that the current standard norms of vitamin B_{12} levels are too low. One Japanese study states the normal limits as 500–1,300 pg/mL. Range of vitamin B12 levels in humans is considered as normal: >300 pg/mL; moderate deficiency: 201–300 pg/mL; and severe deficiency: <201 pg/mL.

Serum vitamin B_{12} tests results are in pg/mL (picograms/milliliter) or pmol/L (picomoles/liter). The laboratory reference ranges for these units are similar, since the molecular weight of B_{12} is approximately 1000, the difference between mL and L. Thus: 550 pg/mL = 400 pmol/L.

Serum homocysteine and methylmalonic acid levels are considered more reliable indicators of B_{12} deficiency than the concentration of B_{12} in blood. The levels of these substances are high in B_{12} deficiency and can be helpful if the diagnosis is unclear.

Routine monitoring of methylmalonic acid levels in urine is an option for people who may not be getting enough dietary B_{12}, as a rise in methylmalonic acid levels may be an early indication of deficiency.

If nervous system damage is suspected, B_{12} analysis in cerebrospinal fluid is possible, though such an invasive test should be considered only if blood testing is inconclusive.

The Schilling test has been largely supplanted by tests for antiparietal cell and intrinsic factor antibodies.

Effect of Folic Acid

The National Institutes of Health has found that "Large amounts of folic acid can mask the damaging effects of vitamin B_{12} deficiency by correcting the megaloblastic anemia caused by vitamin B_{12} deficiency without correcting the neurological damage that also occurs", there are also indications that "high serum folate levels might not only mask vitamin B_{12} deficiency, but could also exacerbate the anemia and worsen the cognitive symptoms associated with vitamin B_{12} deficiency". Due to the fact that in the United States legislation has required enriched flour to contain folic acid to reduce cases of fetal neural-tube defects, consumers may be ingesting more than they realize. To counter the masking effect of B_{12} deficiency the NIH recommends "folic acid intake from fortified food and supplements should not exceed 1,000 μg daily in healthy adults." Most importantly, B_{12} deficiency needs to be treated with B_{12} repletion. Limiting folic acid will not counter the irrevocable neurological damage that is caused by untreated B_{12} deficiency.

Treatment

B_{12} can be supplemented by pill or injection and appear to be equally effective in those with low levels due to absorption problems.

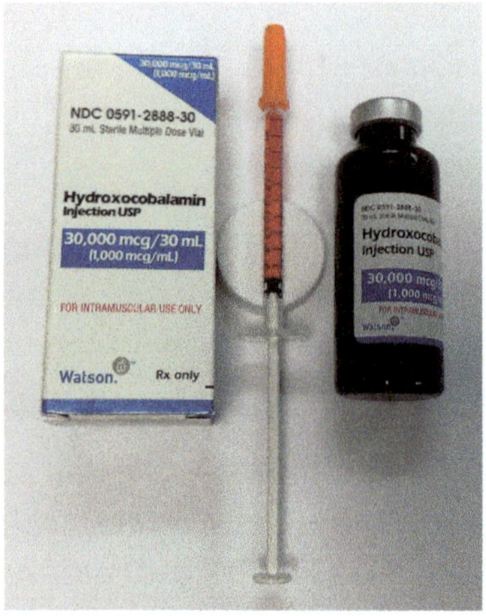

Hydroxocobalamin injection is a clear red liquid solution of hydroxocobalamin.

When large doses are given by mouth its absorption does not rely on the presence of intrinsic factor or an intact ileum. Generally 1 to 2 mg daily is required as a large dose. Even pernicious anemia can be treated entirely by the oral route. These supplements carry such large doses of the vitamin that 1% to 5% of high oral doses of free crystalline B_{12} is absorbed along the entire intestine by passive diffusion.

Epidemiology

In the developing world the deficiency is very widespread, with significant levels of deficiency in Africa, India, and South and Central America. This is theorized to be due to low intakes of animal products, particularly among the poor.

B_{12} deficiency is more common in the elderly. This is because B_{12} absorption decreases greatly in the presence of atrophic gastritis, which is common in the elderly.

The 2000 Tufts University study found no correlation between eating meat and differences in B_{12} serum levels, likely due to a combination of fortified foods and B_{12} absorption disorders.

Veterinary Medicine

Ruminants, such as cows and sheep, absorb B_{12} produced by bacteria in their guts. For gut bacteria of ruminants to produce B_{12} the animal must consume sufficient amounts of cobalt in order for B_{12} to be synthesized. In the early 20th century during the development for farming of the North Island Volcanic Plateau of New Zealand, cattle suffered from what was termed "bush sickness". It was discovered that the volcanic soils lacked the cobalt salts essential for the cattle food chain. The "coast disease" of sheep in the Ninety Mile Desert of the Southeast of South Australia in the 1930s was found to originate in nutritional deficiencies of the trace elements, cobalt and copper. The cobalt deficiency was overcome by the development of "cobalt bullets", dense pellets of cobalt oxide mixed with clay given orally for lodging in the animal's rumen.

Mineral Deficiency

Mineral deficiency is a lack of dietary minerals, the micronutrients that are needed for an organism's proper health. The cause may be a poor diet, impaired uptake of the minerals that are consumed or a dysfunction in the organism's use of the mineral after it is absorbed. These deficiencies can result in many disorders including anemia and goitre. Examples of mineral deficiency include, zinc deficiency, iron deficiency, and magnesium deficiency.

Fluorine Deficiency

Fluoride or fluorine deficiency is a disorder which may cause increased dental caries (or tooth decay, is the breakdown of dental tissues by the acidic products released by the "bacterial fermentation of dietary carbohydrates.") and possibly osteoporosis (a bone disorder which leads to a decrease in bone mass, and an increase in bone fragility), due to a lack of fluoride in the diet; however, there are anti-osteoporotic functional food ingredients that can help decrease the risk of osteoporosis fractures. In terms of dietary sources, fish and tea are considered natural sources of fluoride, as well as tap water that has been fluoridated. The extent to which the condition truly exists, and its relationship to fluoride poisoning has given rise to some controversy. Fluorine is not considered to be an essential nutrient, but the importance of fluorides for preventing tooth decay is well-recognized, although the effect is predominantly topical. Prior to 1981, the effect of fluorides was thought to be largely systemic and preeruptive, requiring ingestion. Fluoride is considered essential in the development and maintenance of teeth by the American Dental Hygienists' Association. Fluoride is also essential as it incorporates into the teeth to form and harden teeth enamels so that the teeth are more acid resistant as well as more resistant to cavity forming bacteria. Caries-inhibiting effects of fluoride were first seen in 1902 when fluoride in high concentrations was found to stain teeth and prevent tooth decay.

Fluoride salts, particularly sodium fluoride (NaF), are used in the treatment and prevention of osteoporosis. Symptoms such as fractured hips in the elderly or brittle and weak bones are caused due to fluorine deficiency in the body. Fluoride stimulates bone formation and increases bone density, however bone with excess fluoride content has an abnormal structure resulting in increased fragility. Thus fluoride therapy results in large increases in bone mineral density but the effect on fracture rates, while positive, is small.

Disputes over the essentiality of fluorine date back to the 19th century, when fluorine was observed in teeth and bones. In 1973 a trial found reduced reproduction in mice fed fluorine-deficient diets, but a subsequent investigation determined that this was due to reduced iron absorption.

Role of Fluoride

Fluoride has proven to be an essential element with preventative and protective properties. Fluoride is capable of combating and working against tooth decay and increases resistance to the "demineralisation of tooth enamel during attack by acidic bacterias". While essential for all individuals, it is significant for children, as when ingested, the fluoride is incorporated into their developing enamel. This in turn causes their teeth to become less prone to decay. Therefore, a relationship can be formulated, in that the more fluoride entering the body, the overall decline in the rate of decay.

Sources of Fluoride

Fluorine is one of the most common and rich elements to exist within the Earth's crust. It is most commonly found in its ion form, or additionally as inorganic or organic fluorides. There are a number of sources of fluoride, these include:

Water

In Australia fluoride occurs naturally within water supplies, at a concentration of approximately 0.1 mg/L. However, this number varies amongst different populations, as specific fluoridated communities exceed this amount, ranging from 0.6-1.0 mg/L of fluoride present. The process of incorporating more fluoride into water systems is an affordable mechanism that can provide many beneficial effects in the long term.

Dentrifices

Fluoride toothpaste came into production in the 1890s, after its benefits were investigated. This product has become available to most industrialised countries, and within Australia accounts for "90% of total toothpaste purchased".

Fluoride Supplements

Fluoride supplements were first recognised and highly suggested by health professionals, in areas where the practice of fluoridating water was not accepted. Such mechanisms are recommended for individuals, primarily children (whom of which are at a greater risk of caries) in low-fluoride areas. Supplements can be in various forms including tablets, drops or lozenges, and have proven to greatly decrease the case and rate of tooth decay.

Iodine Deficiency

Iodine deficiency is a lack of the trace element iodine, an essential nutrient in the diet. It may result in a goiter, sometimes as an endemic goiter as well as cretinism due to untreated congenital hypothyroidism, which results in developmental delays and other health problems. Iodine deficiency is an important public health issue as it is a preventable cause of intellectual disability.

Iodine is an essential dietary mineral; the thyroid hormones thyroxine and triiodothyronine contain iodine. In areas where there is little iodine in the diet, typically remote inland areas where no marine foods are eaten, iodine deficiency is common. It is also common in mountainous regions of the world where food is grown in iodine-poor soil.

Prevention includes adding small amounts of iodine to table salt, a product known as *iodized salt*. Iodine compounds have also been added to other foodstuffs, such as flour, water and milk, in areas of deficiency. Seafood is also a well known source of iodine.

Iodine deficiency resulting in goiter occurs in 187 million people globally as of 2010 (2.7% of the population). It resulted in 2700 deaths in 2013 up from 2100 deaths in 1990.

Signs and Symptoms

Goitre

A low amount of thyroxine (one of the two thyroid hormones) in the blood, due to lack of dietary iodine to make it, gives rise to high levels of thyroid stimulating hormone (TSH), which stimulates the thyroid gland to increase many biochemical processes; the cellular growth and proliferation can result in the characteristic swelling or hyperplasia of the thyroid gland, or goiter. In mild iodine deficiency, levels of triiodiothyronine (T_3) may be elevated in the presence of low levels of levothyroxine, as the body converts more of the levothyroxine to triiodothyronine as a compensation. Some such patients may have a goiter, without an elevated TSH. The introduction of iodized salt since the early 1900s has eliminated this condition in many affluent countries; however, in Australia, New Zealand, and several European countries, iodine deficiency is a significant public health problem. It is more common in third-world nations. Public health initiatives to lower the risk of cardiovascular disease have resulted in lower discretionary salt use at the table. Additionally, there is a trend towards consuming more processed foods in western countries. The noniodized salt used in these foods means that people are less likely to obtain iodine from adding salt during cooking.

Goiter is said to be endemic when the prevalence in a population is > 5%, and in most cases goiter can be treated with iodine supplementation. If goiter is untreated for around five years, however, iodine supplementation or thyroxine treatment may not reduce the size of the thyroid gland because the thyroid is permanently damaged.

Cretinism

Iodine deficiency is one of the leading causes of preventable mental handicaps worldwide, producing typical reductions in IQ of 10 to 15 IQ points. It has been speculated that deficiency of iodine and other micronutrients may be a possible factor in observed differences in IQ between ethnic groups.

Cretinism is a condition associated with iodine deficiency and goiter, commonly characterised by mental deficiency, deafness, squint, disorders of stance and gait and stunted growth due to hypothyroidism. Paracelsus was the first to point out the relation between goitrous parents and their mentally disabled children.

As a result of restricted diet, isolation, intermarriage, etc., as well as low iodine content in their food, children often had peculiar stunted bodies and retarded mental faculties, a condition later known to be associated with thyroid hormone deficiency. Diderot, in his 1754 *Encyclopédie*, described these patients as "crétins". In French, the term "crétin des Alpes" also became current, since the condition was observed in remote valleys of the Alps in particular. The word *cretin* appeared in English in 1779.

While reporting recent progress towards overcoming iodine-deficiency disorders worldwide, *The Lancet* noted: "According to World Health Organization, in 2007, nearly 2 billion individuals had insufficient iodine intake, a third being of school age." A conclusion was made that the single most preventable cause of intellectual disability is that of iodine deficiency.

Fibrocystic Breast Changes

There is preliminary evidence that iodine deficiency enhances the sensitivity of breast tissue to estrogen. In rats treated with estradiol, iodine deficiency has been shown to lead to changes similar to benign breast changes that are reversible by increased iodine in the diet. In a few studies, iodine supplementation had beneficial effects (such as reducing the presence of breast cyst, fibrous tissue plaques and breast pain) in women with fibrocystic breast changes.

Protective effects of iodine on breast cancer have been postulated from epidemiologic evidence and described in animal models. In view of the antiproliferative properties of iodine in breast tissue, molecular iodine supplementation has been suggested as an adjuvant in breast cancer therapy.

Deficient Populations

In areas where there is little iodine in the diet, typically remote inland areas and semi-arid equatorial climates where no marine foods are eaten, iodine deficiency gives rise to hypothyroidism, symptoms of which are extreme fatigue, goiter, mental slowing, depression, weight gain, and low basal body temperatures.

Iodine deficiency is the leading cause of preventable mental retardation, a result which occurs primarily when babies or small children are rendered hypothyroidic by a lack of the element. The addition of iodine to table salt has largely eliminated this problem in the wealthier nations, but as of March 2006, iodine deficiency remained a serious public health problem in the developing world.

Iodine deficiency is also a problem in certain areas of Europe. In Germany it has been estimated to cause a billion dollars in health care costs per year. A modelling analysis suggests universal iodine supplementation for pregnant women in England may save £199 (2013 UK pounds) to the health service per pregnant woman and save £4476 per pregnant woman in societal costs.

Risk Factors

Following is a list of potential risk factors that may lead to iodine deficiency:

1. Low dietary iodine
2. Selenium deficiency
3. Pregnancy
4. Exposure to radiation
5. Increased intake/plasma levels of goitrogens, such as calcium
6. Gender (higher occurrence in women)
7. Smoking tobacco
8. Alcohol (reduced prevalence in users)
9. Oral contraceptives (reduced prevalence in users)
10. Perchlorates
11. Thiocyanates
12. Age (for different types of iodine deficiency at different ages)

In the U.S., the use of iodine has decreased over concerns of overdoses since mid-20th century, and the iodine antagonists bromine, perchlorate and fluoride have become more ubiquitous. In particular, around 1980 the practice of using potassium iodate as dough conditioner in bread and baked goods was gradually replaced by the use of other conditioning agents such as bromide.

Pathophysiology

Iodine accounts for 65% of the molecular weight of T4 and 59% of the T3. 15–20 mg of iodine is concentrated in thyroid tissue and hormones, but 70% of the body's iodine is distributed in other tissues, including mammary glands, eyes, gastric mucosa, choroid plexus, arterial walls, the cervix, and salivary glands. In the cells of these tissues, iodide enters directly by sodium-iodide symporter (NIS).

- *Venturi S, Guidi A, Venturi M (1996). "[Extrathyroid iodine deficiency disorders: what is the real iodine requirement?]".". Le Basi Razionali della Terapia. 16: 267–275.*
- *Pellerin P (1961). "La tecnique d'autoradiographie anatomique a la temperature de l'azote liquide". Path Biol. 232 (9): 233–252.*
- Byeong-Cheol Ahn (2011). "Physiologic and False Positive Pathologic Uptakes on Radioiodine Whole Body Scan".

Diagnosis

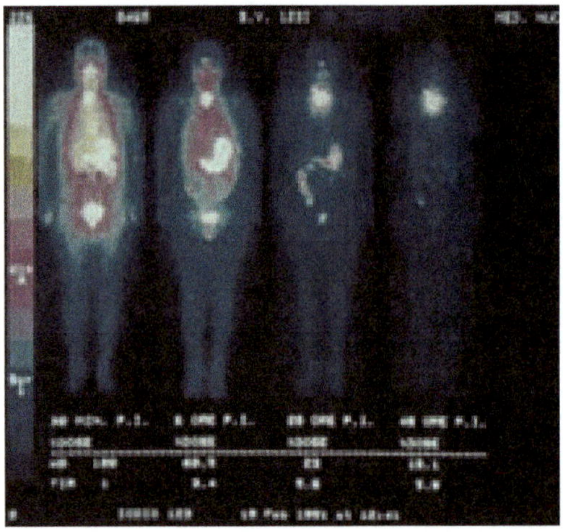

Sequence of 123-iodide human scintiscans after an intravenous injection, (from left) after 30 minutes, 20 hours, and 48 hours. A high and rapid concentration of radio-iodide is evident in the periencephalic and cerebrospinal fluid (left), salivary glands, oral mucosa and the stomach. In the thyroid gland, I-concentration is more progressive, also in the reservoir (from 1% after 30 minutes, to 5.8% after 48 hours, of the total injected dose.

If a 24-hour urine collection is not practical, a random urine iodine-to-creatinine ratio can alternatively be used. However, the 24-hour test is found to be more reliable.

A general idea of whether a deficiency exists can be determined through a functional iodine test in the form of an iodine skin test. In this test, the skin is painted with an iodine solution: if the iodine patch disappears quickly, this is taken as a sign of iodine deficiency. However, no accepted norms exist on the expected time interval for the patch to disappear, and in persons with dark skin color the disappeance of the patch may be difficult to assess. If a urine test is taken shortly after, the results may be altered due to the iodine absorbed previously in a skin test.

Treatment

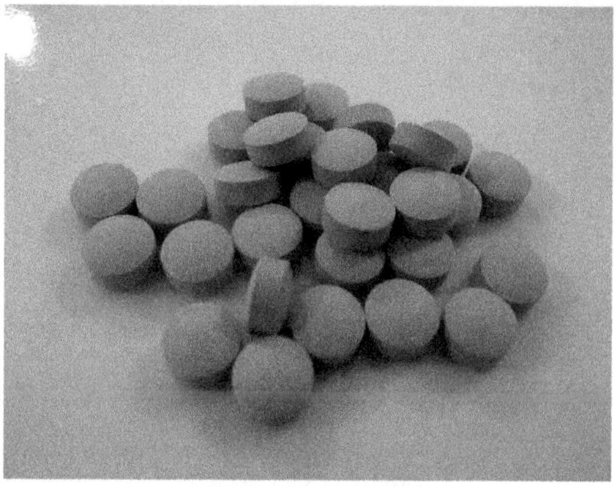

Iodine supplements

Iodine deficiency is treated by ingestion of iodine salts, such as found in food supplements. Mild cases may be treated by using iodized salt in daily food consumption, or drinking more milk, or eating egg yolks, and saltwater fish. For a salt and/or animal product restricted diet, sea vegetables (kelp, hijiki, dulse, nori (found in sushi)) may be incorporated regularly into a diet as a good source of iodine.

The recommended daily intake of iodine for adult women is 150–300 µg for maintenance of normal thyroid function; for men it is somewhat less at 150 µg.

However, too high iodine intake, for example due to overdosage of iodine supplements, can have toxic side effects. It can lead to hyperthyroidism and consequently high blood levels of thyroid hormones (hyperthyroxinemia). In case of extremely high single-dose iodine intake, typically a short-term suppression of thyroid function (Wolff–Chaikoff effect) occurs. Persons with pre-existing thyroid disease, elderly persons, fetuses and neonates, and patients with other risk factors are at a higher risk of experiencing iodine-induced thyroid abnormalities. In particular, in persons with goiter due to iodine deficiency or with altered thyroid function, a form of hyperthyroidism called Jod-Basedow phenomenon can be triggered even at small or single iodine dosages, for example as a side effect of administration of iodine-containing contrast agents. In some cases, excessive iodine contributes to a risk of autoimmune thyroid diseases (Hashimoto's thyroiditis and Graves' disease).

Epidemiology

Iodine deficiency resulting in goiter occurs 187 million people globally as of 2010 (2.7% of the population). Certain areas of the world, due to natural deficiency and unavailability of iodine, are severely affected by iodine deficiency, which affects approximately two billion people worldwide. It is particularly common in the Western Pacific, South-East Asia and Africa. Among other nations affected by iodine deficiency, China and Kazakhstan have begun taking action, while Russia has not. Successful campaigns for the adoption of the use of iodized salt require education of salt producers and sellers and a communication campaign directed at the public. The cost of adding iodine to salt is negligible—"Only a few cents a ton."

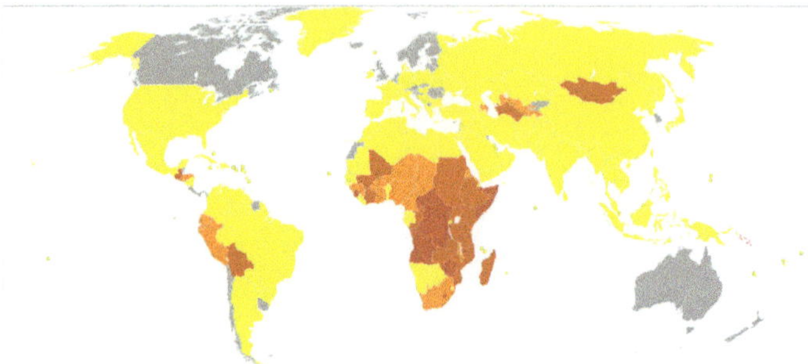

Deaths due to iodine deficiency per million persons in 2012

0-0 1-1 2-3 4-18

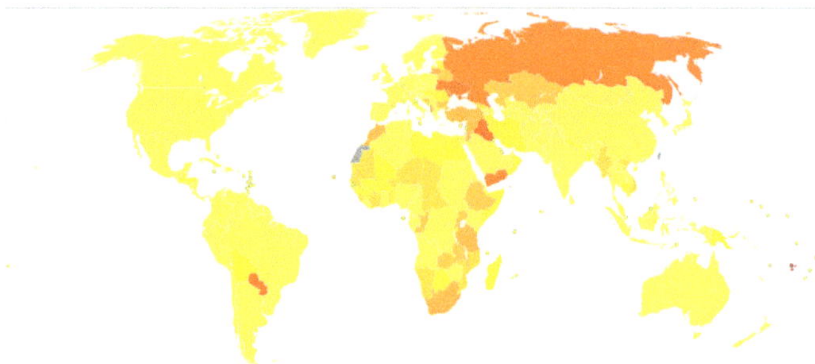

Disability-adjusted life year for iodine deficiency per 100,000 inhabitants in 2004.

no data	150-200	350-400
<50	200-250	400-450
50-100	250-300	450-500
100-150	300-350	500-750
		>750

Iodine deficiency has largely been confined to the developing world for several generations, but reductions in salt consumption and changes in dairy processing practices eliminating the use of iodine-based disinfectants have led to increasing prevalence of the condition in Australia and New Zealand in recent years. A proposal to mandate the use of iodized salt in most commercial breadmaking was adopted there in October, 2009. In a study of the United Kingdom published in 2011, almost 70% of test subjects were found to be iodine deficient. The study's authors suggested an investigation regarding "evidence-based recommendations for iodine supplementation".

It is well known that micronutrient deficiencies change the development of intelligence and iodine is no exception. Lacking in iodine during human development causes a fall, in average, of 12 IQ points in China.

Scientists James Feyrer, Dimitra Politi, and David N. Weil have found in the U.S. that the proliferation of iodized salt increased IQ by 15 points in some areas. Journalist Max Nisen has stated that, with this type of salt becoming popular, that "the aggregate effect has been extremely positive."

In iodine deficient or mildly iodine deficient areas in Europe, iodine deficiency is frequent during pregnancy despite the widespread use of iodised salt, posing risks to the neurodevelopment of foetuses. In one study performed in a midly iodine-deficient area, iodine deficiency was found to be present in more than half of breastfeeding women; in contrast, the majority of their newborns had iodine excess, mostly due to neonatal exposure to iodine-containing disinfectants. A 2014 meta-analysis found that iodine supplementation "improves some maternal thyroid indices and may benefit aspects of cognitive function in school-age children, even in marginally iodine-deficient areas."

Prognosis

With iodine supplementation, goiters caused by iodine deficiency decrease in size in very young children and pregnant women. Generally, however, long-standing goiters caused by iodine deficiency respond with only small amounts of shrinkage after iodine supplementation, and patients are at risk for developing hyperthyroidism. Following the adoption of iodised salt in the United States in 1924 there was a gradual increase in average intelligence of 1 standard deviation, 15 points in iodine-deficient areas, 3.5 points nationally, but also an increase in deaths of older people in iodine-deficient areas due to hyperthyroidism.

Research

In view of large-scale epidemiological studies of iodine levels in populations, a method of capillary electrophoresis with UV detection of iodine has been proposed.

Zinc Deficiency

Zinc deficiency can occur in soil, plants, and animals. In animals, including humans, it is defined either qualitatively as insufficient zinc to meet the needs of the body and thereby causing clinical manifestations, or quantitatively as a serum zinc level below the normal range; however, serum zinc is not a reliable biomarker for zinc status in humans, as a decrease in serum concentration is only detectable after long-term or severe depletion. Novel zinc biomarkers, such as the erythrocyte LA:DGLA ratio, have shown promise in pre-clinical and clinical trials and are being developed to more accurately detect dietary zinc deficiency. Zinc deficiency affects about 2.2 billion people around the world.

Zinc deficiency in humans results from reduced dietary intake, inadequate absorption, increased loss, or increased use. The most common cause is reduced dietary intake; as much as 25% of the world's population is at risk. Increasing the amount of zinc in the soil and thus in crops is an effective preventative measure. Zinc plays an essential role in numerous biochemical pathways. It affects many organ systems, including the skin, gastrointestinal tract, central nervous system, and immune, skeletal, and reproductive systems. A lack of zinc thus has numerous manifestations, the most common of which are an increased rates of diarrhea, pneumonia, and malaria.

Classification

Zinc deficiency affects about 2.2 billion people around the world. Zinc deficiency can be classified as acute, as may occur during prolonged inappropriate zinc-free total parenteral nutrition; or chronic, as may occur in dietary deficiency or inadequate absorption. Lactation, alcoholism, old age, and metabolic disorders are associated with zinc deficiency in adults.

Signs and Symptoms

Skin, Nails and Hair

Zinc deficiency may manifest as acne, eczema, xerosis (dry, scaling skin), seborrheic dermatitis, or alopecia (thin and sparse hair). There may also be impaired wound healing.

Mouth

Zinc deficiency can manifest as non-specific oral ulceration, stomatitis, or white tongue coating. Rarely it can cause angular cheilitis (sores at the corners of the mouth) and burning mouth syndrome.

Vision, Smell and Taste

Severe zinc deficiency may disturb the sense of smell and taste. Night blindness may be a feature of severe zinc deficiency, however most reports of night blindness and abnormal dark adaptation in humans with zinc deficiency have occurred in combination with other nutritional deficiencies (e.g. vitamin A).

Immune System

Impaired immune function in people with zinc deficiency can lead to the development of respiratory, gastrointestinal, or other infections, e.g., pneumonia. The levels of inflammatory cytokines (e.g., IL-1β, IL-2, IL-6, and TNF-α) in blood plasma are affected by zinc deficiency and zinc supplementation produces a dose-dependent response in the level of these cytokines. During inflammation, there is an increased cellular demand for zinc and impaired zinc homeostasis from zinc deficiency is associated with chronic inflammation.

Diarrhea

Zinc deficiency contributes to an increased incidence and severity of diarrhea.

Appetite

Zinc deficiency may lead to loss of appetite or anorexia nervosa. The use of zinc in the treatment of anorexia has been advocated since 1979 by Bakan. At least 15 clinical trials have shown that zinc improved weight gain in anorexia. A 1994 trial showed that zinc doubled the rate of body mass increase in the treatment of anorexia nervosa. Deficiency of other nutrients such as tyrosine, tryptophan and thiamine could contribute to this phenomenon of "malnutrition-induced malnutrition".

Cognitive Function and Hedonic Tone

Cognitive functions, such as learning and hedonic tone, are impaired with zinc deficiency. Moderate and more severe zinc deficiencies are associated with behavioral abnormalities, such as irritability, lethargy, and depression (e.g., involving anhedonia). Zinc supplementation produces a rapid and dramatic improvement in hedonic tone (i.e., general level of happiness or pleasure) under these circumstances. Zinc supplementation has been reported to improve symptoms of ADHD and depression.

Psychological Disorders

Plasma zinc levels have been alleged to be associated with many psychological disorders. An increasing amount of evidence suggests that zinc deficiency could play a role in depression. Zinc supplementation may be an effective treatment in major depression.

Growth

Zinc deficiency in children can cause delayed growth and has been claimed to be the cause of stunted growth in one third of the world's population.

During Pregnancy

Zinc deficiency during pregnancy can negatively affect both the mother and fetus. Animal studies indicate that maternal zinc deficiency can upset both the sequencing and efficiency of the birth process. An increased incidence of difficult and prolonged labor, hemorrhage, uterine dystocia and placental abruption has been documented in zinc deficient animals. These effects may be mediated by the defective functioning of estrogen via the estrogen receptor, which contains a zinc finger protein. A review of pregnancy outcomes in women with acrodermatitis enteropathica, reported that out of every seven pregnancies, there was one abortion and two malfunctions, suggesting the human fetus is also susceptible to the teratogenic effects of severe zinc deficiency. However, a review on zinc supplementation trials during pregnancy did not report a significant effect of zinc supplementation on neonatal survival.

Zinc deficiency can interfere with many metabolic processes when it occurs during infancy and childhood, a time of rapid growth and development when nutritional needs are high. Low maternal zinc status has been associated with less attention during the neonatal period and worse motor functioning. In some studies, supplementation has been associated with motor development in very low birth weight infants and more vigorous and functional activity in infants and toddlers.

Testosterone Production

Zinc is required to produce testosterone. Thus, zinc deficiency can lead to reduced circulating testosterone, hypogonadism and delayed puberty.

Causes

Dietary Deficiency

A diet which is high in phytate containing whole grains, high in foods grown in zinc deficient soil, or high in processed foods containing little or no zinc can result in zinc deficiency. Conservative estimates suggest that 25% of the world's population is at risk of zinc deficiency.

In the U.S., the Recommended Dietary Allowance (RDA) is 8 mg/day for women and 11 mg/day for men. The following table summarizes most of the foods with significant quantities of zinc, listed in order of quantity per serving, unfortified. Note that all of the top 10 entries are meat, beans, or nuts. The recommended intake per day of zinc is 15 mg for adults and children over the age of four.

Food	mg in one serving	Percentage of recommended daily intake
Oysters, cooked, breaded and fried, 3 ounces (about 5 average sized oysters)	74.0	493%
Beef chuck roast, braised, 3 ounces	7.0	47%
Crab, Alaska king, cooked, 3 ounces	6.5	43%
Beef patty, broiled, 3 ounces	5.3	35%
Cashews, dry roasted, 3 ounces	4.8	33%
Lobster, cooked, 3 ounces	3.4	23%
Pork chop, loin, cooked, 3 ounces	2.9	19%
Baked beans, canned, plain or vegetarian, ½ cup	2.9	19%
Almonds, dry roasted, 3 ounces	2.7	18%
Chicken, dark meat, cooked, 3 ounces	2.4	16%
Yogurt, fruit, low fat, 8 ounces	1.7	11%

Chickpeas, cooked, ½ cup	1.3	9%
Cheese, Swiss, 1 ounce	1.2	8%
Oatmeal, instant, plain, prepared with water, 1 packet	1.1	7%
Milk, low-fat or non fat, 1 cup	1.0	7%
Kidney beans, cooked, ½ cup	0.9	6%
Chicken breast, roasted, skin removed, ½ breast	0.9	6%
Cheese, cheddar or mozzarella, 1 ounce	0.9	6%
Peas, green, frozen, cooked, ½ cup	0.5	3%
Flounder or sole, cooked, 3 ounces	0.3	2%

Inadequate Absorption

Acrodermatitis enteropathica is an inherited deficiency of the zinc carrier protein ZIP4 resulting in inadequate zinc absorption. It presents as growth retardation, severe diarrhea, hair loss, skin rash (most often around the genitalia and mouth) and opportunistic candidiasis and bacterial infections.

Numerous small bowel diseases which cause destruction or malfunction of the gut mucosa enterocytes and generalized malabsorption are associated with zinc deficiency.

Increased Loss

Exercising, high alcohol intake, and diarrhea all increase loss of zinc from the body. Changes in intestinal tract absorbability and permeability due, in part, to viral, protozoal, or bacteria pathogens may also encourage fecal losses of zinc.

Increased Utilization

Exercising, childhood growth, and pregnancy all increase utilization.

Chronic Disease

The mechanism of zinc deficiency in some diseases has not been well defined; it may be multifactorial.

Wilson's disease, sickle cell disease, chronic kidney disease, chronic liver disease have all been associated with zinc deficiency. It can also occur after bariatric surgery, mercury exposure and tartrazine.

Although marginal zinc deficiency is often found in depression, low zinc levels could either be a cause or a consequence of mental disorders and their symptoms.

Mechanism

As biosystems are unable to store zinc, regular intake is necessary. Excessively low zinc intake can lead to zinc deficiency, which can negatively impact an individual's health. The mechanisms for the clinical manifestations of zinc deficiency are best appreciated by recognizing that zinc functions in the body in three areas: catalytic, structural, and regulatory. Zinc (Zn) is only common in its +2 oxidative state, where it typically coordinates with tetrahedral geometry. It is important in maintaining basic cellular functions such as DNA replication, RNA transcription, cell division and cell activations. However, having too much or too little zinc can cause these functions to be compromised.

In its catalytic role, zinc is a critical component of the catalytic site of hundreds of kinds of different metalloenzymes in each human being. In its structural role, zinc coordinates with certain protein domains, facilitating protein folding and producing structures such as 'zinc fingers'. In its regulatory role, zinc is involved in the regulation of nucleoproteins and the activity of various inflammatory cells. For example, zinc regulates the expression of metallothionein, which has multiple functions, such as intracellular zinc compartmentalization and antioxidant function. Thus zinc deficiency results in disruption of hundreds of metabolic pathways, causing numerous clinical manifestations, including impaired growth and development, and disruption of reproductive and immune function.

Pra1 (pH regulated antigen 1) is a candida albicans protein that scavenges host zinc.

Prevention

Five interventional strategies can be used:

- Adding zinc to soil, called agronomic biofortification, which both increases crop yields and provides more dietary zinc.
- Adding zinc to food, called fortification.
- Adding zinc rich foods to diet. The foods with the highest concentration of zinc are proteins, especially animal meats, the highest being oysters. Per ounce, beef, pork, and lamb contain more zinc than fish. The dark meat of a chicken has more zinc than the light meat. Other good sources of zinc are nuts, whole grains, legumes, and yeast. Although whole grains and cereals are high in zinc, they also contain chelating phytates which bind zinc and reduce its bioavailability.
- Oral repletion via tablets (e.g. zinc gluconate) or liquid (e.g. zinc acetate). Oral zinc supplementation in healthy infants more than six months old has been shown to reduce the duration of any subsequent diarrheal episodes by about 11 hours.
- Oral repletion via multivitamin/mineral supplements containing zinc gluconate, sulfate, or acetate. It is not clear whether one form is better than another. Zinc is also found in some cold lozenges, nasal sprays, and nasal gels.

Epidemiology

Severe zinc deficiency is rare, and is mainly seen in persons with acrodermatitis enteropathica, a severe defect in zinc absorption due to a congenital deficiency in the zinc carrier protein ZIP4 in the enterocyte. Mild zinc deficiency due to reduced dietary intake is common. Conservative estimates suggest that 25% of the world's population is at risk of zinc deficiency. Zinc deficiency is thought to be a leading cause of infant mortality.

Providing micronutrients, including zinc, to humans is one of the four solutions to major global problems identified in the Copenhagen Consensus from an international panel of economists.

History

Significant historical events related to zinc deficiency began in 1869 when zinc was first discovered to be essential to the growth of an organism (Aspergillus Niger). In 1929 Lutz measured zinc in numerous human tissues using the dithizone technique and estimated total body zinc in a 70 kg man to be 2.2 grams. Zinc was found to be essential to the growth of rats in 1933. In 1939 beriberi patients in China were noted to have decreased zinc levels in skin and nails. In 1940 zinc levels in a series of autopsies found it to be present in all tissues examined. In 1942 a study showed most zinc excretion was via the feces. In 1950 a normal serum zinc level was first defined, and found to be 17.3–22.1 micromoles/liter. In 1956 cirrhotic patients were found to have low serum zinc levels. In 1963 zinc was determined to be essential to human growth, three enzymes requiring zinc as a cofactor were described, and a report was published of a 21-year-old Iranian man with stunted growth, infantile genitalia, and anemia which were all reversed by zinc supplementation. In 1972 fifteen Iranian rejected army inductees with symptoms of zinc deficiency were reported: all responded to zinc. In 1973 the first case of acrodermatitis enteropathica due to severe zinc deficiency was described. In 1974 the National Academy of Sciences declared zinc to be an essential element for humans and established a recommended daily allowance. In 1978 the Food and Drug Administration required zinc to be in total parenteral nutrition fluids. In the 1990s there was increasing attention on the role of zinc deficiency in childhood morbidity and mortality in developing countries. In 2002 the zinc transporter protein ZIP4 was first identified as the mechanism for absorption of zinc in the gut across the basolateral membrane of the enterocyte. By 2014 over 300 zinc containing enzymes have been identified, as well as over 1000 zinc containing transcription factors.

Soils and Crops

Soil zinc is an essential micronutrient for crops. Almost half of the world's cereal crops are deficient in zinc, leading to poor crop yields. Many agricultural countries around the world are affected by zinc deficiency. In China, zinc deficiency occurs on around half of the agricultural soils, affecting mainly rice and maize. Areas with zinc deficient soils are often regions with widespread zinc deficiency in humans. A basic knowledge of the dynamics of zinc in soils, understanding of the uptake and transport of zinc in crops and characterizing the response of crops to zinc deficiency are essential steps in achieving sustainable solutions to the problem of zinc deficiency in crops and humans.

Biofortification

Soil and foliar application of zinc fertilizer can effectively increase grain zinc and reduce the phytate:zinc ratio in grain. People who eat bread prepared from zinc enriched wheat have a significant increase in serum zinc.

Zinc fertilization not only increases zinc content in zinc deficient crops, it also increases crop yields. Balanced crop nutrition supplying all essential nutrients, including zinc, is a cost effective management strategy. Even with zinc-efficient varieties, zinc fertilizers are needed when the available zinc in the topsoil becomes depleted.

Plant breeding can improve zinc uptake capacity of plants under soil conditions with low chemical availability of zinc. Breeding can also improve zinc translocation which elevates zinc content in edible crop parts as opposed to the rest of the plant.

Central Anatolia, in Turkey, was a region with zinc-deficient soils and widespread zinc deficiency in humans. In 1993, a research project found that yields could be increased by 6 to 8-fold and child nutrition dramatically increased through zinc fertilization. Zinc was added to fertilizers. While the product was initially made available at the same cost, the results were so convincing that Turkish farmers significantly increased the use of the zinc-fortified fertilizer (1 percent of zinc) within a few years, despite the repricing of the products to reflect the added value of the content. Nearly ten years after the identification of the zinc deficiency problem, the total amount of zinc-containing compound fertilizers produced and applied in Turkey reached a record level of 300,000 tonnes per annum. It is estimated that the economic benefits associated with the application of zinc fertilizers on zinc deficient soils in Turkey is around US$100 million per year. Zinc deficiency in children has been dramatically reduced.

Hypocalcaemia

Hypocalcaemia, also spelled hypocalcemia, is low calcium levels in the blood serum. The normal range is 2.1–2.6 mmol/L (8.8–10.7 mg/dL, 4.3–5.2 mEq/L) with levels less than 2.1 mmol/L defined as hypocalcemia. Mildly low levels that develop slowly often have no symptoms. Otherwise symptoms may include numbness, muscle spasms, seizures, confusion, or cardiac arrest.

Common causes include hypoparathyroidism and vitamin D deficiency. Others causes include kidney failure, pancreatitis, calcium channel blocker overdose, rhabdomyolysis, tumor lysis syndrome, and medications such as bisphosphonates. Diagnosis should generally be confirmed with a corrected calcium or ionized calcium level. Specific changes may be seen on an electrocardiogram (ECG).

Initial treatment for severe disease is with intravenous calcium chloride and possibly magnesium sulfate. Other treatments may include vitamin D, magnesium, and calcium supplements. If due to hypoparathyroidism, hydrochlorothiazide, phosphate binders, and a low salt diet may also be recommended. About 18% of people who are in hospital have hypocalcemia.

Signs and Symptoms

The neuromuscular symptoms of hypocalcemia are caused by a positive bathmotropic effect due to the decreased interaction of calcium with sodium channels. Since calcium blocks sodium channels and inhibits depolarization of nerve and muscle fibers, reduced calcium lowers the threshold for depolarization. The symptoms can be recalled by the mnemonic "CATs go numb" - Convulsions, Arrhythmias, Tetany, and numbness/parasthesias in the hands and feet and around the mouth.

- Petechiae which appear as on-off spots, then later become confluent, and appear as purpura (larger bruised areas, usually in dependent regions of thc body).
- Oral, perioral and acral paresthesias, tingling or 'pins and needles' sensation in and around the mouth and lips, and in the extremities of the hands and feet. This is often the earliest symptom of hypocalcaemia.
- Carpopedal and generalized tetany (unrelieved and strong contractions of the hands, and in the large muscles of the rest of the body) are seen.
- Latent tetany
  - Trousseau sign of latent tetany (eliciting carpal spasm by inflating the blood pressure cuff and maintaining the cuff pressure above systolic)
  - Chvostek's sign (tapping of the inferior portion of the cheekbone will produce facial spasms)
- Tendon reflexes are hyperactive
- Life-threatening complications
  - Laryngospasm
  - Cardiac arrhythmias
- Effects on cardiac output
  - Negative chronotropic effect, or a decrease in heart rate.
  - Negative inotropic effect, or a decrease in contractility

- ECG changes include the following:
    - o Intermittent QT prolongation, or intermittent prolongation of the QTc (corrected QT interval) on the EKG (electrocardiogram) is noted. The implications of intermittent QTc prolongation predisposes to life-threatening cardiac electrical instability (and this is therefore a more critical condition than constant QTc prolongation). This type of electrical instability puts the patient at high risk of torsades de pointes, a specific type of ventricular tachycardia which appears on an EKG (or ECG) as something which looks a bit like a sine wave with a regularly increasing and decreasing amplitude. (Torsades de pointes can cause death, unless the patient can be medically or electrically cardioverted and returned to a normal cardiac rhythm.)

Causes

Hypoparathyroidism is a common cause of hypocalcemia. Calcium is tightly regulated by the parathyroid hormone (PTH). In response to low calcium levels, PTH induces the kidneys to reabsorb calcium, the kidneys to increase production of calcitriol (the active form of vitamin D) thereby increasing intestinal absorption of calcium, and the bones to release calcium. These actions lead to a re-balance in the blood calcium levels. However, in the setting of absent, decreased, or ineffective PTH hormone, the body loses this regulatory function, and hypocalcemia ensues. Hypoparathyroidism is commonly due to surgical destruction of the parathyroid glands via parathyroidectomy or neck dissection for head and neck cancers. Hypoparathyroidism may also be due to autoimmune destruction of the glands.

- Eating disorders
- Prolonged vomiting (e.g. with a viral illness)
- Exposure to mercury, including infantile acrodynia
- Excessive dietary magnesium, as with supplementation.
- Excessive dietary zinc, as with supplementation (causes rapid hypocalcemia).
- Prolonged use of medications/laxatives containing magnesium
- Chelation therapy for metal exposure, particularly EDTA
- Osteoporosis treatment or preventive agents, such as bisphosphonates and denosumab.
- Agents for the treatment of hypercalcemia, such as Calcitonin.
- Chronic kidney failure
- Absent active vitamin D

- Decreased dietary intake
- Decreased sun exposure
- Defective Vitamin D metabolism
    - Anticonvulsant therapy
    - Vitamin-D dependent rickets, type I

- Ineffective active vitamin D
    - Intestinal malabsorption
    - Vitamin-D dependent rickets, type II
- Pseudohypoparathyroidism
- Severe acute hyperphosphataemia
- Tumour lysis syndrome
- Acute kidney failure
    - Rhabdomyolysis (initial stage)
- Exposure to hydrofluoric acid
- As a complication of pancreatitis
- Alkalosis, often caused by hyperventilation
    - As blood plasma hydrogen ion concentration decreases, caused by respiratory or metabolic alkalosis, the concentration of freely ionized calcium, the biologically active component of blood calcium, decreases. Because a portion of both hydrogen ions and calcium are bound to serum albumin, when blood becomes alkalotic, the bound hydrogen ions dissociate from albumin, freeing up the albumin to bind with more calcium and thereby decreasing the freely ionized portion of total serum calcium. For every 0.1 increase in pH, ionized calcium decreases by about 0.05 mmol/L. This hypocalcaemia related to alkalosis is partially responsible for the cerebral vasoconstriction that causes the lightheadedness, fainting, and paraesthesia often seen with hyperventilation.
    - Tetany may also be seen with this condition.
- Neonatal hypocalcemia
    - Very low birth weight (less than 1500 grams)
    - Gestational age less than 32 weeks

Mechanism

Physiologically, blood calcium is tightly regulated within a narrow range for proper cellular processes. Calcium in the blood exists in three primary states: bound to proteins (mainly albumin), bound to anions such as phosphate and citrate, and as free (unbound) ionized calcium. Only the ionized calcium is physiologically active. Normal blood calcium level is between 8.5 to 10.5 mg/dL (2.12 to 2.62 mmol/L) and that of ionized calcium is 4.65 to 5.25 mg/dL (1.16 to 1.31 mmol/L).

Diagnosis

Because a significant portion of calcium is bound to albumin, any alteration in the level of albumin will affect the measured level of calcium. A corrected calcium level based on the albumin level is: Corrected calcium (mg/dL) = measured total Ca (mg/dL) + 0.8 * (4.0 - serum albumin [g/dL]). Another way to determine the calcium level is to measure directly the ionized calcium level.

Management

- Intravenous calcium gluconate 10% can be administered, or if the hypocalcaemia is severe, calcium chloride is given instead. This is only appropriate if the hypocalcemia is acute and has occurred over a relatively short time frame. But if the hypocalcemia has been severe and chronic, then this regimen can be fatal, because there is a degree of acclimatization that occurs. The neuromuscular excitability, cardiac electrical instability, and associated symptoms are then not cured or relieved by prompt administration of corrective doses of calcium, but rather exacerbated. Such rapid administration of calcium would result in effective over correction – symptoms of hypercalcemia would follow.
- However, in either circumstance, maintenance doses of both calcium and vitamin-D (often as 1,25-$(OH)_2$-D_3, i.e. calcitriol) are often necessary to prevent further decline.

Selenium Deficiency

Selenium deficiency is relatively rare in healthy well-nourished individuals. Few cases in humans have been reported.

Causes

It can occur in patients with severely compromised intestinal function, those undergoing total parenteral nutrition, those who have had gastrointestinal bypass surgery, and also in persons of advanced age (i.e., over 90).

People dependent on food grown from selenium-deficient soil may be at risk for deficiency.

For some time now, it has been reported in medical literature that a pattern of side-effects possibly associated with cholesterol-lowering drugs (e.g., statins) may resemble the pathology of selenium deficiency.

Reference Ranges

In the US, the Dietary Reference Intake for adults is 55 µg/day. In the UK it is 75 µg/day for adult males and 60 µg/day for adult females. 55 µg/day recommendation is based on full expression of plasma glutathione peroxidase. Selenoprotein P is a better indicator of selenium nutritional status, and full expression of it would require more than 66 µg/day.

Signs and Symptoms

Selenium deficiency in combination with Coxsackievirus infection can lead to Keshan disease, which is potentially fatal. Selenium deficiency also contributes (along with iodine deficiency) to Kashin-Beck disease. The primary symptom of Keshan disease is myocardial necrosis, leading to weakening of the heart. Kashin-Beck disease results in atrophy, degeneration and necrosis of cartilage tissue. Keshan disease also makes the body more susceptible to illness caused by other nutritional, biochemical, or infectious diseases.

Selenium is also necessary for the conversion of the thyroid hormone thyroxine (T4) into its more active counterpart, triiodothyronine, and as such a deficiency can cause symptoms of hypothyroidism, including extreme fatigue, mental slowing, goiter, cretinism, and recurrent miscarriage.

Epidemiology and Prevention

These diseases are most common in certain parts of China where the intake is low because the soil is extremely deficient in selenium. Studies in Jiangsu Province of China have indicated a reduction in the prevalence of these diseases by taking selenium supplements. In Finland, selenium salts are added to chemical fertilizers, as a way to increase selenium in soils.

In Non-human Animals

In some regions (e.g. much of the northeastern and northwestern US and adjacent Canada, and the southeastern US), selenium deficiency in some animal species is common unless supplementation is carried out. Selenium deficiency is responsible (either alone or together with vitamin E deficiency) for many of the cases of WMD ("white muscle disease"), evidenced at slaughter or during necropsy by whitish appearance of striated muscle tissue due to bleaching by peroxides and hydroperoxides. Although this degenerative disease can occur in foals, pigs and other animal species, ruminants are particularly susceptible. In general, absorption of dietary selenium is lower in ruminants than in non-ruminants, and is lower from forages than from grain. Sheep are more susceptible than cattle to WMD, and goats are more susceptible than sheep. Because of selenium's role in certain peroxidases (converting hydroperoxides to alcohols) and because of the antioxidant role of vitamin E (preventing hydroperoxide formation), a low level of Se can be somewhat (but not wholly) compensated by a high level of vitamin E. (In the animal, localization of peroxidases and vitamin E differs, partly because of the fat-solubility of vitamin E.) Some studies have indicated that about 0.12 or 0.23 mg Se per kg of dry matter intake may be sufficient for avoiding Se deficiency in sheep in some circumstances. However, somewhat higher Se intake may be required for avoidance of WMD where certain legumes are consumed. The cyanogenic glycosides in some white clover (*Trifolium repens*) varieties may influence the Se requirement, presumably because of cyanide from the aglycone released by glucosidase activity in the rumen and inactivation of glutathione peroxidases by the effect of absorbed cyanide on the glutathione moiety.

In areas where selenium deficiency in livestock is a concern, selenium (as selenite) may be supplemented in feed. In some countries, e.g. the US and Canada, such supplementation is regulated. Neonate ruminants at risk of WMD may be administered both Se and vitamin E by injection; some of the WMD myopathies respond only to Se, some only to vitamin E, and some to either.

Thiamine Deficiency

Thiamine deficiency commonly presents subacutely and can lead to metabolic coma and death. A lack of thiamine can be caused by malnutrition, a diet high in thiaminase-rich foods (raw freshwater fish, raw shellfish, ferns) and/or foods high in anti-thiamine factors (tea, coffee, betel nuts) and by grossly impaired nutritional status associated with chronic diseases, such as alcoholism, gastrointestinal diseases, HIV-AIDS, and persistent vomiting. It is thought that many people with diabetes have a deficiency of thiamine and that this may be linked to some of the complications that can occur.

Well-known syndromes caused by thiamine deficiency include beriberi, Wernicke-Korsakoff syndrome, and optic neuropathy.

Thiamine derivatives and thiamine-dependent enzymes are present in all cells of the body, thus a thiamine deficiency would seem to adversely affect all of the organ systems. However, the nervous system is particularly sensitive to thiamine deficiency, because of its dependence on oxidative metabolism.

Beriberi

Beriberi is a neurological and cardiovascular disease. The three major forms of the disorder are dry beriberi, wet beriberi, and infantile beriberi. A fourth form, gastrointestinal beriberi, was recognized in 2004.

- *Dry beriberi* is characterized principally by peripheral neuropathy consisting of symmetric impairment of sensory, motor, and reflex functions affecting distal more than proximal limb segments and causing calf muscle tenderness.

However, it has been recently recognized that peripheral neuropathy (tingling or numbness in the extremities) due to thiamine deficiency could also present with axonal neuropathy (partial paralysis or sensory loss). Peripheral neuropathy can present with subacute motor axonal neuropathy mimicking Guillain–Barré syndrome; or as a large fibre proprioceptive central-peripheral axonal neuropathy presenting as a subacute sensory ataxia.

- *Wet beriberi* is associated with mental confusion, muscular atrophy, edema, tachycardia, cardiomegaly, and congestive heart failure in addition to peripheral neuropathy

- *Infantile beriberi* occurs in infants breast-fed by thiamin-deficient mothers (who may show no sign of thiamine deficiency). Infants may manifest cardiac, aphonic, or pseudomeningitic forms of the disorder. Infants with cardiac beriberi frequently exhibit a loud piercing cry, vomiting, and tachycardia. Convulsions are not uncommon, and death may ensue if thiamine is not administered promptly.

- *Gastrointestinal beriberi* is associated with nausea, vomiting, abdominal pain, and lactic acidosis.

Following thiamine treatment, rapid improvement occurs, in general, within 24 hours. Improvements of peripheral neuropathy may require several months of thiamine treatment.

Alcoholic Brain Disease

Nerve cells and other supporting cells (such as glial cells) of the nervous system require thiamine. Alcoholism can reduce the body's ability to transport, metabolise and store thiamine. Examples of neurologic disorders that are linked to alcohol abuse include Wernicke's encephalopathy (WE), Korsakoff's syndrome (alcohol amnestic disorder), Wernicke–Korsakoff syndrome as well as varying degrees of cognitive impairment.

Wernicke's encephalopathy is the most frequently encountered manifestation of thiamine deficiency in Western society, though it may also occur in patients with impaired nutrition from other causes, such as gastrointestinal disease, those with HIV-AIDS, and with the injudicious administration of parenteral glucose or hyperalimentation without adequate B-vitamin supplementation. This is a striking neuro-psychiatric disorder characterized by paralysis of eye movements, abnormal stance and gait, and markedly deranged mental function.

Korsakoff's syndrome is, in general, considered to occur with deterioration of brain function in patients initially diagnosed with WE. This is an amnestic-confabulatory syndrome characterized by retrograde and anterograde amnesia, impairment of conceptual functions, and decreased spontaneity and initiative.

Alcoholics may have thiamine deficiency because of the following:

- Inadequate nutritional intake: Alcoholics tend to intake less than the recommended amount of thiamine.
- Decreased uptake of thiamine from the GI tract: Active transport of thiamine into enterocytes is disturbed during acute alcohol exposure.
- Liver thiamine stores are reduced due to hepatic steatosis or fibrosis.
- Impaired thiamine utilization: Magnesium, which is required for the binding of thiamine to thiamine-using enzymes within the cell, is also deficient due to chronic alcohol consumption. The inefficient utilization of any thiamine that does reach the cells will further exacerbate the thiamine deficiency.
- Ethanol *per se* inhibits thiamine transport in the gastrointestinal system and blocks phosphorylation of thiamine to its cofactor form (ThDP).

Following improved nutrition and the removal of alcohol consumption, some impairments linked with thiamine deficiency are reversed, in particular poor brain functionality, although in more severe cases, Wernicke–Korsakoff syndrome leaves permanent damage.

Optic Neuropathy

Optic neuropathy can also occur in thiamine deficiency and is characterized by bilateral visual loss, cecocentral scotomas and impaired colour perception. The ophthalmological findings usually can show a bilateral oedema of the optic disk in the acute phase, followed by a bilateral optic atrophy.

Genetic Diseases

Genetic diseases of thiamine transport are rare but serious. Thiamine responsive megaloblastic anemia (TRMA) with diabetes mellitus and sensorineural deafness is an autosomal recessive disorder caused by mutations in the gene SLC19A2, a high affinity thiamine transporter. TRMA patients do not show signs of systemic thiamine deficiency, suggesting redundancy in the thiamine transport system. This has led to the discovery of a second high-affinity thiamine transporter, SLC19A3. Leigh disease (subacute necrotising encephalomyelopathy) is an inherited disorder that affects mostly infants in the first years of life and is invariably fatal. Pathological similarities between Leigh disease and WE led to the hypothesis that the cause was a defect in thiamine metabolism. One of the most consistent findings has been an abnormality of the activation of the pyruvate dehydrogenase complex.

Mutations in the SLC19A3 gene have been linked to Biotin-Thiamine Responsive Basal Ganglia Disease which is treated with pharmacological doses of thiamine and biotin, another B vitamin.

Other disorders in which a putative role for thiamine has been implicated include subacute necrotising encephalomyelopathy, opsoclonic cerebellopathy (a paraneoplastic syndrome), and Nigerian seasonal ataxia. In addition, several inherited disorders of ThDP-dependent enzymes have been reported, which may respond to thiamine treatment.

Diagnosis

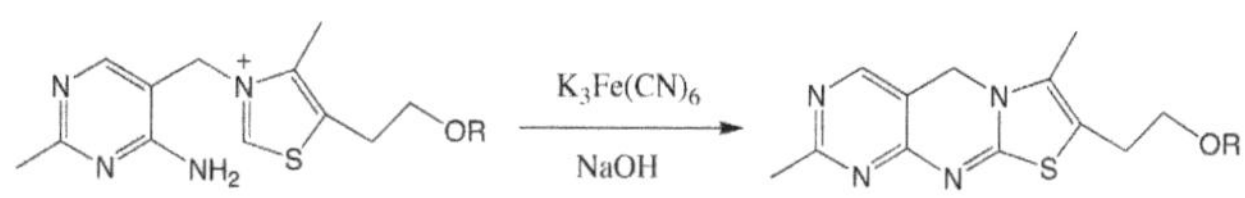

R = H	Thiamine	Thiochrome
R = PO_3^{2-}	ThMP	ThcMP
R = $P_2O_6^{3-}$	ThDP	ThcDP
R = $P_3O_9^{4-}$	ThTP	ThcTP
R = $P_3O_8^{3-}$-adenosine	AThTP	AThcTP

Oxidation of thiamine derivatives to fluorescent thiochromes by potassium ferricyanide under alkaline conditions

A positive diagnosis test for thiamine deficiency can be ascertained by measuring the activity of the enzyme transketolase in erythrocytes (Erythrocyte Transketolase Activation Assay). Thiamine, as well as its phosphate derivatives, can also be detected directly in whole blood, tissues, foods, animal feed, and pharmaceutical preparations following the conversion of thiamine to fluorescent thiochrome derivatives (Thiochrome Assay) and separation by high-performance liquid chromatography (HPLC). In recent reports, a number of Capillary Electrophoresis (CE) techniques and in-capillary enzyme reaction methods have emerged as potential alternative techniques for the determination and monitoring of thiamine in samples. The normal thiamine concentration in EDTA-blood is about 20-100 μg/l.

Other Animals

Poultry

As most feedstuffs used in poultry diets contain enough quantities of vitamins to meet the requirements in this species, deficiencies in this vitamin do not occur with commercial diets. This was, at least, the opinion in the 1960s.

Mature chickens show signs 3 weeks after being fed a deficient diet. In young chicks, it can appear before 2 weeks of age.

Onset is sudden in young chicks. There is anorexia and an unsteady gait. Later on, there are locomotor signs, beginning with an apparent paralysis of the flexor of the toes. The characteristic position is called "stargazing", meaning a chick "sitting on its hocks and the head in opisthotonos".

Response to administration of the vitamin is rather quick, occurring a few hours later.

Differential diagnosis include riboflavin deficiency and avian encephalomyelitis. In riboflavin deficiency, the "curled toes" is a characteristic symptom. Muscle tremor is typical of avian encephalomyelitis. A therapeutic diagnosis can be tried by supplementing thiamine only in the affected bird. If the animals do not respond in a few hours, thiamine deficiency can be excluded.

Ruminants

Polioencephalomalacia (PEM) is the most common thiamine deficiency disorder in young ruminant and nonruminant animals. Symptoms of PEM include a profuse, but transient, diarrhea, listlessness, circling movements, star gazing or opisthotonus (head drawn back over neck), and muscle tremors. The most common cause is high-carbohydrate feeds, leading to the overgrowth of thiaminase-producing bacteria, but dietary ingestion of thiaminase (e.g., in bracken fern), or inhibition of thiamine absorption by high sulfur intake are also possible. Another cause of PEM is *Clostridium sporogenes* or *Bacillus aneurinolyticus* infection. These bacteria produce thiaminases that will cause an acute thiamine deficiency in the affected animal.

Wild Birds and Fish

Thiamine deficiency has been identified as the cause of a paralytic disease affecting wild birds in the Baltic Sea area dating back to 1982. In this condition, there is difficulty in keeping the wings folded along the side of the body when resting, loss of the ability to fly and voice, with eventual paralysis of the wings and legs and death. It affects primarily 0.5–1 kg sized birds such as the herring gull (*Larus argentatus*), common starling (*Sturnus vulgaris*) and common eider (*Somateria mollissima*). Researches noted, "Because the investigated species occupy a wide range of ecological niches and positions in the food web, we are open to the possibility that other animal classes may suffer from thiamine deficiency as well."

In the counties of Blekinge and Skåne (south-most Sweden) mass deaths of especially herring gull but also other species has been observed since the early 2000s. More recently, species of other classes seems to be affected. High mortality of salmon (*Salmo salar*) in the river Mörrumsån is reported, and the last years mammals like Eurasian

Elk (*Alces alces*) has suffered death in unusual high number. Lack of thiamine is the common denominator where analysis is done. The County Administrative Board of Blekinge did in April 2012 find the situation so alarming that they asked the Swedish government to set up a closer investigation.

References

- Weick MT (1967). “A history of rickets in the United States”. The American Journal of Clinical Nutrition. 20 (11): 1234–41. PMID 4862158
- Latham, Michael E. (1997). Human Nutrition in the Developing World (Fao Food and Nutrition Paper). Food & Agriculture Organization of the United. ISBN 92-5-103818-X
- “Dietary Supplement Fact Sheet: Vitamin D”. National Institutes of Health. Archived from the original on 2007-09-10. Retrieved 2007-09-10
- Schoenen J, Jacquy J, Lenaerts M (Feb 1998). “Effectiveness of high-dose riboflavin in migraine prophylaxis. A randomized controlled trial”. Neurology. 50 (2): 466–70. PMID 9484373. doi:10.1212/wnl.50.2.466
- Lips P (2007). “Vitamin D status and nutrition in Europe and Asia”. The Journal of Steroid Biochemistry and Molecular Biology. 103 (3–5): 620–5. PMID 17287117. doi:10.1016/j.jsbmb.2006.12.076
- edited by Lindsay Allen ... (2006). Guidelines on Food Fortification With Micronutrients. Geneva: World Health Organization. ISBN 92-4-159401-2
- Cherniack; Levis; Troen (2008). “Hypovitaminosis D: a widespread epidemic”. Geriatrics. Retrieved 14 April 2015
- Ink, S. L.; Henderson, L. M. (1984). “Vitamin B_6 metabolism”. Annu. Rev. Nutr. 4 (1): 455–470. PMID 6380540. doi:10.1146/annurev.nu.04.070184.002323
- Holick MF (November 2005). “The vitamin D epidemic and its health consequences”. The Journal of Nutrition. 135 (11): 2739S–48S. PMID 16251641
- Ross AC, Taylor CL, Yaktine AL, Del Valle HB (2011). Dietary Reference Intakes for Calcium and Vitamin D. Washington, D.C: National Academies Press. ISBN 0-309-16394-3
- Kingsbury, Kathleen (2008-10-13). “Kids Aren’t Getting Enough Vitamin D”. Time Health & Science. Time Inc. Retrieved 15 November 2008
- Dalton, K.; Dalton, M. J. T. (Jul 1987). “Characteristics of pyridoxine overdose neuropathy syndrome”. Act. Neurol. Scand. 76 (1): 8–11. PMID 3630649. doi:10.1111/j.1600-0404.1987.tb03536.x
- Xu L.; Lee M.; Jeyabalan A.; Roberts J.M. (2014). “The relationship of hypovitaminosis D and IL-6 in preeclampsia”. American Journal of Obstetrics and Gynaecology. 210 (2): 149–149
- Page, C.; Blake, D.; Winyard, P.G. (1995). Immunopharmacology of Free Radical Species. Elsevier Science. p. 136. ISBN 9780080534541. Retrieved 12 April 2015
- Wortsman, J., Matsuoka, L. Y., Chen, T. C., Lu, Z., & Holick, M. F, J, Y, C, Z & F (2000). “Decreased bioavailability of vitamin D in obesity”. The American Journal of Clinical Nutrition. Retrieved 15 April 2015
- Desai, A; Sequeira, JM; Quadros, EV (July 2016). “The metabolic basis for developmental disorders due to defective folate transport.”. Biochimie. 126: 31–42. PMID 26924398. doi:10.1016/j.biochi.2016.02.012

- DN Amarapurka MD, ND Patel MD (September 2004). “Gastric Antral Vascular Ectasia Syndrome”. Journal of The Association of Physcians of India. 52: 757
- Hamilton, Richart (2015). Tarascon Pocket Pharmacopoeia 2015 Deluxe Lab-Coat Edition. Jones & Bartlett Learning. p. 230. ISBN 9781284057560
- Office of Dietary Supplements. “Vitamin E Professional Fact Sheet”. National Institutes of Health. Retrieved 14 August 2010
- 'Vilela';'Nunes', ‘Pedro’; ‘Teresa’ (2011). “Osteoporosis International”. Neuroradiology. 53: 185–189. doi:10.1007/s00234-011-0925-4
- Sethi NK, Robilotti E, Sadan Y (2005). “Neurological Manifestations Of Vitamin B-12 Deficiency”. The Internet Journal of Nutrition and Wellness. 2 (1). doi:10.5580/5a9
- Handbook of Behavior, Food and Nutrition, edited by Victor R. Preedy, Ronald Ross Watson, Colin R. Martin, Springer Science & Business Media, 15 Apr 2011, Ch.153, p.2428, ISBN 9780387922713

4

Effects of Malnutrition

Malnutrition is the deficiency or surplus of nutrients in the body. The effects of malnutrition are Wernicke-Korsakoff syndrome, stunted growth, wasting, rickets, anemia, pellagra and beriberi. The aspects elucidated in this chapter are of vital importance, and provide a better understanding of the effects of malnutrition.

Wernicke–Korsakoff Syndrome

Wernicke–Korsakoff syndrome (WKS) is the combined presence of Wernicke's encephalopathy (WE) and Korsakoff's syndrome. Due to the close relationship between these two disorders, people with either are usually diagnosed with WKS, as a single syndrome.

The cause of the disorder is thiamine (vitamin B_1) deficiency, which can cause a range of disorders including beriberi, Wernicke's encephalopathy, and Korsakoff's psychosis. These disorders may manifest together or separately. WKS is usually secondary to alcohol abuse. It mainly causes vision changes, ataxia and impaired memory.

Wernicke's encephalopathy and WKS are most commonly seen in people who are alcoholic, and only 20% of cases are identified before death. This failure in diagnosis of WE and thus treatment of the disease leads to death in approximately 20% of cases, while 75% are left with permanent brain damage associated with WKS. Of those affected, 25% require long-term institutionalization in order to receive effective care.

Signs and Symptoms

The syndrome is a combined manifestation of two namesake disorders, Wernicke's encephalopathy and Korsakoff's psychosis. It involves an acute Wernicke-encephalopathy phase, followed by the development of a chronic Korsakoff's syndrome phase.

Wernicke's Encephalopathy

WE is characterized by the presence of a triad of symptoms;

1. Ocular disturbances (ophthalmoplegia)
2. Changes in mental state (confusion)
3. Unsteady stance and gait (ataxia)

This triad of symptoms results from a deficiency in vitamin B_1 which is an essential co-enzyme. The aforementioned changes in mental state occur in approximately 82% of patients' symptoms of which range from confusion, apathy, inability to concentrate, and a decrease in awareness of the immediate situation they are in. If left untreated, WE can lead to coma or death. In about 29% of patients, ocular disturbances consist of nystagmus and paralysis of the lateral rectus muscles or other muscles in the eye. A smaller percentage of patients experience a decrease in reaction time of the pupils to light stimuli and swelling of the optic disc which may be accompanied by retinal hemorrhage. Finally, the symptoms involving stance and gait occur in about 23% of patients and result from dysfunction in the cerebellum and vestibular system. Other symptoms that have been present in cases of WE are stupor, low blood pressure (hypotension), elevated heart rate (tachycardia), as well as hypothermia, epileptic seizures and a progressive loss of hearing.

Interestingly, about 19% of patients have none of the symptoms in the classic triad at first diagnosis of WE; however, usually one or more of the symptoms develops later as the disease progresses.

Korsakoff's Syndrome

KS is described as an acute onset of severe memory impairment without any dysfunction in intellectual abilities. The DSM IV lists the following criteria for the diagnosis of Korsakoff's Syndrome:

1. anterograde amnesia
2. Variable presentation of retrograde amnesia

One of:

1. Aphasia
2. Apraxia
3. Agnosia
4. A deficit in executive functions

In addition, the DSM-IV indicates that normal activities and function will be impaired by the memory deficits and that the experience of amnesia must occur outside of times where the individual is in a state of delirium, intoxification, or withdrawal. The criteria for diagnosis also maintain that there must be evidence that the amnesia is caused by the use of alcohol.

Despite the assertion that Korsakoff's syndrome must be caused by the use of alcohol, there have been several cases where it has developed from other instances of thiamine deficiency resulting from gross malnutrition due to conditions such as; stomach cancer, anorexia nervosa, and gastrectomy.

Cognitive Effects

Several cases have been documented where Wernicke-Korsakoff Syndrome has been seen on a large scale. In 1947, 52 cases of WKS were documented in a prisoner of war hospital in Singapore where the prisoner's diets included less than 1 mg of thiamine per day. Such cases provide an opportunity to gain an understanding of what effects this syndrome has on cognition. In this particular case, cognitive symptoms included insomnia, anxiety, difficulties in concentration, loss of memory for the immediate past, and gradual degeneration of mental state; consisting of confusion, confabulation, and hallucinations. In other cases of WKS, cognitive effects such as severely disrupted speech, giddiness, and heavy headedness have been documented. In addition to this, it has been noted that some patients displayed an inability to focus, and the inability of others to catch patients' attention.

In a study conducted in 2003 by Brand et al. on the cognitive effects of WKS, the researchers used a neuropsychological test battery which included tests of intelligence, speed of information processing, memory, executive function and cognitive estimation. They found that patients suffering from WKS showed impairments in all aspects of this test battery but most noticeably, on the cognitive estimation tasks. This task required subjects to estimate a physical quality such as size, weight, quantity or time (i.e. What is the average length of a shower?), of a particular item. Patients with WKS performed worse than normal control participants on all of the tasks in this category. The patients found estimations involving time to be the most difficult, whereas quantity was the easiest estimation to make. Additionally, the study included a category for classifying "bizarre" answers, which included any answer that was far outside of the normal range of expected responses. WKS patients did give answers that could fall into such a category and these included answers such as 15s or 1 hour for the estimated length of a shower, or 4 kg or 15 tonnes as the weight of a car.

Memory Deficits

As mentioned previously, the amnesic symptoms of WKS include both retrograde and anterograde amnesia. The retrograde deficit has been demonstrated through an inability of WKS patients to recall or recognize information for recent public events. The anterograde memory loss is demonstrated through deficits in tasks that involve encoding and then recalling lists of words and faces, as well as semantic learning tasks. WKS patients have also demonstrated difficulties in preservation as evidenced by a deficit in performance on the Wisconsin Card Sorting Test. The retrograde amnesia that accompanies WKS can extend as far back as twenty to thirty years, and there is generally a temporal gradient seen, where earlier memories are recalled better than more recent memories. It has been widely accepted that the critical structures that lead to the memory impairment in WKS are the mammillary bodies, and the thalamic regions. Despite the aforementioned memory deficits, non-declarative memory functions appear to be intact in WKS patients. This has been demonstrated through measures that assess perceptual priming.

Other studies have shown deficits in recognition memory and stimulus-reward associative functions in patients with WKS. The deficit in stimulus-reward functions was demonstrated by Oscar-Berman and Pulaski who presented patients with reinforcements for certain stimuli but not others, and then required the patients to distinguish the rewarded stimuli from the non-rewarded stimuli. WKS patients displayed significant deficits in this task. The researchers were also successful in displaying a deficit in recognition memory by having patients make a yes/no decision as to whether a stimulus was familiar (previously seen) or novel (not previously seen). The patients in this study also showed a significant deficit in their ability to perform this task.

Confabulation

People with WKS often show confabulation, spontaneous confabulation being seen more frequently than provoked confabulation. Spontaneous confabulations refer to incorrect memories that the patient holds to be true, and may act on, arising spontaneously without any provocation. Provoked confabulations can occur when a patient is cued to give a response, this may occur in test settings. The spontaneous confabulations viewed in WKS are thought to be produced by an impairment in source memory, where they are unable to remember the spatial and contextual information for an event, and thus may use irrelevant or old memory traces to fill in for the information that they cannot access. It has also been suggested that this behaviour may be due to executive dysfunction where they are unable to inhibit incorrect memories or because they are unable to shift their attention away from an incorrect response.

Causes

WKS is usually found in chronic alcoholics. Wernicke–Korsakoff syndrome results from thiamine deficiency. It is generally agreed that Wernicke's encephalopathy results from severe acute deficiency of thiamine (vitamin B_1), whilst Korsakoff's psychosis is a chronic neurologic sequela of Wernicke's encephalopathy. The metabolically active form of thiamine is thiamine pyrophosphate, which plays a major role as a cofactor or coenzyme in glucose metabolism. The enzymes which are dependent on thiamine pyrophosphate are associated with the citric acid cycle (also known as the Krebs cycle), and catalyze the oxidation of pyruvate, α-ketoglutarate and branched chain amino acids. Thus, anything that encourages glucose metabolism will exacerbate an existing clinical or sub-clinical thiamine deficiency.

As stated above, Wernicke–Korsakoff syndrome in the United States is usually found in malnourished chronic alcoholics, though it is also found in patients who undergo prolonged intravenous (IV) therapy without vitamin B_1 supplementation, gastric stapling, intensive care unit (ICU) stays or hunger strikes. In some regions, physicians have observed thiamine deficiency brought about by severe malnutrition, particularly in diets consisting mainly of polished rice, which is thiamine-deficient. The resulting nervous system ailment is called beriberi. In individuals with sub-clinical thiamine deficiency, a large dose of glucose (either as sweet food, etc. or glucose infusion) can precipitate the onset of overt encephalopathy.

Wernicke–Korsakoff syndrome in alcoholics particularly is associated with atrophy/infarction of specific regions of the brain, especially the mamillary bodies. Other regions include the anterior region of the thalamus (accounting for amnesic symptoms), the medial dorsal thalamus, the basal forebrain, the median and dorsal raphe nuclei, and the cerebellum.

One as-yet-unreplicated study has associated susceptibility to this syndrome with a hereditary deficiency of transketolase, an enzyme that requires thiamine as a coenzyme.

Post-gastrectomy

The fact that gastrointestinal surgery can lead to the development of WKS was demonstrated in a study that was completed on three patients who recently undergone a gastrectomy. These patients had developed WKS but were not alcoholics and had never suffered from dietary deprivation. WKS developed between 2 and 20 years after the surgery. There were small dietary changes that contributed to the development of WKS but overall the lack of absorption of thiamine from the gastrointestinal tract was the cause. Therefore, it must be ensured that patients who have undergone gastrectomy have a proper education on dietary habits, and carefully monitor their thiamine intake. Additionally, an early diagnosis of WKS, should it develop, is very important.

Alcohol–thiamine Interactions

Strong evidence suggests that ethanol interferes directly with thiamine uptake in the gastrointestinal tract. Ethanol also disrupts thiamine storage in the liver and the transformation of thiamine into its active form. The role of alcohol consumption in the development of WKS has been experimentally confirmed through studies in which rats were subjected to alcohol exposure and lower levels thiamine through a low-thiamine diet. In particular, studies have demonstrated that clinical signs of the neurological problems that result from thiamine deficiency develop faster in rats that have received alcohol and were also deficient in thiamine than rats who did not receive alcohol. In another study, it was found that rats that were chronically fed alcohol had significantly lower liver thiamine stores than control rats. This provides an explanation for why alcoholics with liver cirrhosis have a higher incidence of both thiamine deficiency and WKS.

Pathophysiology

Brain atrophy associated with WKS occurs in the following regions of the brain: the mammillary bodies, the thalamus, the periaqueductal grey, the walls of the 3rd ventricle, the floor of the 4th ventricle, the cerebellum, and the frontal lobe. In addition to the damage seen in these areas there have been reports of damage to cortex, although it was noted that this may be due to the direct toxic effects of alcohol as opposed to thiamine deficiency that has been attributed as the underlying cause of Wernicke-Korsakoff Syndrome.

The amnesia that is associated with this syndrome is a result of the atrophy in the structures of the diencephalon (the thalamus, hypothalamus and mammillary bodies), and is similar to amnesia that is presented as a result of other cases of damage to the medial temporal lobe. It has been argued that the memory impairments can occur as a result of damage along any part of the mammillo-thalamic tract, which explains how WKS can develop in patients with damage exclusively to either the thalamus or the mammillary bodies.

Diagnosis

Diagnosis of Wernicke–Korsakoff syndrome is by clinical impression and can sometimes be confirmed by a formal neuropsychological assessment. Wernicke's encephalopathy typically presents with ataxia and nystagmus, and Korsakoff's psychosis with anterograde and retrograde amnesia and confabulation upon relevant lines of questioning.

Frequently, secondary to thiamine deficiency and subsequent cytotoxic edema in Wernicke's encephalopathy, patients will have marked degeneration of the mamillary bodies. Thiamine (vitamin B_1) is an essential coenzyme in carbohydrate metabolism and is also a regulator of osmotic gradient. Its deficiency may cause swelling of the intracellular space and local disruption of the blood-brain barrier. Brain tissue is very sensitive to changes in electrolytes and pressure and edema can be cytotoxic. In Wernicke's this occurs specifically in the mammillary bodies, medial thalami, tectal plate, and periaqueductal areas. Sufferers may also exhibit a dislike for sunlight and so may wish to stay indoors with the lights off. The mechanism of this degeneration is unknown, but it supports the current neurological theory that the mammillary bodies play a role in various "memory circuits" within the brain. An example of a memory circuit is the Papez circuit.

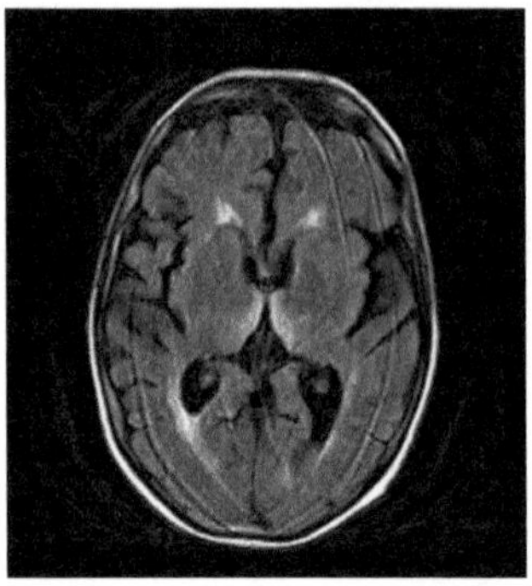

Axial MRI FLAIR image showing hyperintense signal in the mesial dorsal thalami, a common finding in Wernicke encephalopathy. This patient was nearly in coma when IV thiamine was started, he responded moderately well but was left with some Korsakoff type deficits.

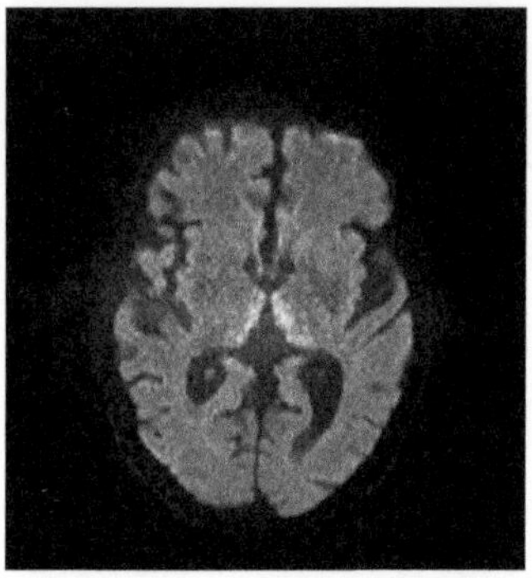

Axial MRI B=1000 DWI image showing hyperintense signal indicative of restricted diffusion in the mesial dorsal thalami.

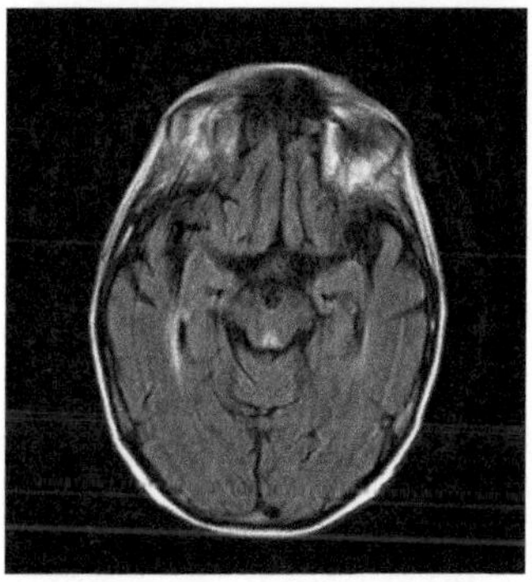

Axial MRI FLAIR image showing hyperintense signal in the periaqueductal gray matter and tectum of the dorsal midbrain.

Treatment

The onset of Wernicke's encephalopathy is considered a medical emergency, and thus thiamine administration should be initiated immediately when the disease is suspected. Prompt administration of thiamine to patients with Wernicke's encephalopathy can prevent the disorder from developing into Wernicke–Korsakoff syndrome, or reduce its severity. Treatment can also reduce the progression of the deficits caused by WKS, but will not completely reverse existing deficits. WKS will continue to be present, at least partially, in 80% of patients. Patients suffering from WE should be given a minimum dose of 500 mg of Thiamine hydrochloride, delivered by infusion over a 30-minute period for two to three days. If no response is seen then treatment should be discontinued but for those patients that do respond, treatment should be continued with a 250 mg dose delivered intravenously or intramuscularly for three to five days unless the patient stops improving. Such prompt administration of thiamine may be a life-saving measure. Banana bags, a bag of intravenous fluids containing vitamins and minerals, is one means of treatment.

Prevention

As described, Korsakoff 's syndrome usually follows or accompanies Wernicke's encephalopathy. If treated quickly, it may be possible to prevent the development of

Korsakoff's syndrome with thiamine treatments. This treatment is not guaranteed to be effective and the thiamine needs to be administered adequately in both dose and duration. A study on Wernicke-Korsakoff's syndrome showed that with consistent thiamine treatment there were noticeable improvements in mental status after only 2–3 weeks of therapy. Thus, there is hope that with treatment Wernicke's encephalopathy will not necessarily progress to WKS.

In order to reduce the risk of developing WKS it is important to limit the intake of alcohol or drink in order to ensure that proper nutrition needs are met. A healthy diet is imperative for proper nutrition which, in combination with thiamine supplements, may reduce the chance of developing WKS. This prevention method may specifically help heavy drinkers who refuse to or are unable to quit.

Epidemiology

Internationally, the prevalence rates of WKS are relatively standard, being anywhere between zero and two percent. Despite this, specific sub-populations seem to have higher prevalence rates including people who are homeless, older individuals (especially those living alone or in isolation), and psychiatric inpatients. Additionally, studies show that prevalence is not connected to alcohol consumption per capita. For example, in France, a country that is well known for its consumption and production of wine, prevalence was only 0.4% in 1994, while Australia had a prevalence of 2.8%.

History

Wernicke's Encephalopathy

Carl Wernicke discovered Wernicke's encephalopathy in 1881. His first diagnosis noted symptoms including paralyzed eye movements, ataxia, and mental confusion. Also noticed were hemorrhages in the gray matter around the third and fourth ventricles and the cerebral aqueduct. Brain atrophy was only found upon post-mortem autopsy. Wernicke believed these hemorrhages were due to inflammation and thus the disease was named polioencephalitis haemorrhagica superior. Later, it was found that Wernicke's encephalopathy and Korsakoff's syndrome are products of the same cause.

Korsakoff's Syndrome

Sergei Korsakoff was a Russian physician after whom the disease "Korsakoff's Syndrome" is named. In the late 1800s Korsakoff was studying long-term alcoholic patients and began to notice a decline in their memory function. At the 13th International Medical Congress in Moscow in 1897, Korsakoff presented a report called: *"On a special form of mental illness combined with degenerative polyneuritis"*. After the presentation of this report the term "Korsakoff's Syndrome" was coined.

Although WE and KS were discovered separately, these two syndromes are usually referred to under one name, Wernicke–Korsakoff syndrome, due to the fact that they are part of the same cause and because the onset of KS usually follows WE if left untreated.

Society and Culture

The British neurologist Oliver Sacks describes case histories of some of his patients with the syndrome in the book *The Man Who Mistook His Wife for a Hat* (1985).

The disease is also portrayed by Patricia Ferreira in the Spanish film *Sé Quién Eres* (*I Know Who You Are*, 2000).

Beriberi

Beriberi refers to symptoms caused by thiamine (vitamin B1) deficiency. Beriberi has conventionally been divided into three separate entities, relating to the body system mainly involved (peripheral nervous system or cardiovascular) or age of person (like infantile). Beriberi is one of several thiamine-deficiency related conditions, which may occur concurrently, including Wernicke's encephalopathy (mainly affecting the central nervous system), Korsakoff's syndrome (amnesia with additional psychiatric manifestations), and Wernicke-Korsakoff syndrome (with both neurologic and psychiatric symptoms).

Historically, beriberi has been common in regions where what is variously referred to as polished or white rice forms a major part of the diet, which has its husk removed to extend its shelf life and palatability but has the side effect of removing the primary source of thiamine. It was not known until the end of the 19th century that polishing rice was associated with beriberi.

Signs and Symptoms

Symptoms of beriberi include weight loss, emotional disturbances, impaired sensory perception, weakness and pain in the limbs, and periods of irregular heart rate. Edema (swelling of bodily tissues) is common. It may increase the amount of lactic acid and pyruvic acid within the blood. In advanced cases, the disease may cause high-output cardiac failure and death. Symptoms may occur concurrently with those of Wernicke's encephalopathy, a primarily neurological thiamine-deficiency related condition.

Beriberi is divided into four categories as follows. The first three are historical and the fourth, gastrointestinal beriberi, was recognized in 2004:

- *Dry beriberi* specially affects the peripheral nervous system

- *Wet beriberi* specially affects the cardiovascular system and other bodily systems
- *Infantile beriberi* affects the children of malnourished mothers
- *Gastrointestinal beriberi* affects the digestive system and other bodily systems

Dry Beriberi

Dry beriberi causes wasting and partial paralysis resulting from damaged peripheral nerves. It is also referred to as endemic neuritis. It is characterized by:

- Difficulty in walking
- Tingling or loss of sensation (numbness) in hands and feet
- Loss of tendon reflexes
- Loss of muscle function or paralysis of the lower legs
- Mental confusion/speech difficulties
- Pain
- Involuntary eye movements (nystagmus)
- Vomiting.

A selective impairment of the large proprioceptive sensory fibers without motor impairment can occur and present as a prominent sensory ataxia, which is a loss of balance and coordination due to loss of the proprioceptive inputs from the periphery and loss of position sense.

Wet Beriberi

Wet beriberi affects the heart and circulatory system. It is sometimes fatal, as it causes a combination of heart failure and weakening of the capillary walls, which causes the peripheral tissues to become edematous. Wet beriberi is characterized by:

- Increased heart rate
- Vasodilation leading to decreased systemic vascular resistance, and high output cardiac failure
- Elevated jugular venous pressure
- Dyspnea (shortness of breath) on exertion
- Paroxysmal nocturnal dyspnea
- Peripheral edema (swelling of lower legs)

Infantile Beriberi

Infantile beriberi usually occurs between two and six months of age in children whose mothers have inadequate thiamine intake. In the acute form, the baby develops dyspnea and cyanosis and soon dies of heart failure. These symptoms may be described in infantile beriberi:

- Hoarseness, where the child makes moves to moan but emits no sound or just faint moans caused by nerve paralysis
- Weight loss, becoming thinner and then marasmic as the disease progresses
- Vomiting
- Diarrhea
- Pale skin
- Edema
- Ill temper
- Alterations of the cardiovascular system, especially tachycardia (rapid heart rate)
- Convulsions occasionally observed in the terminal stages

Gastrointestinal Beriberi

Gastrointestinal beriberi causes abdominal pain. Gastrointestinal beriberi is characterized by:

- Abdominal Pain
- Nausea
- Vomiting
- Lactic Acidosis

Cause

Beriberi may also be caused by shortcomings other than inadequate intake: diseases or operations on the digestive tract, alcoholism, dialysis, genetic deficiencies, etc. All these causes mainly affecting the central nervous system, and provoking the development of what is known as Wernicke's disease or Wernicke's encephalopathy.

Wernicke´s disease is one of the most prevalent neurological or neuropsychiatric diseases. In autopsy series, features of Wernicke lesions are observed in approximately 2% of general cases. Medical record research shows that about 85% had not been diagnosed, although only 19% would be asymptomatic. In children, only 58% were diagnosed. In alcohol abusers, autopsy series showed neurological damages at rates of 12.5% or more. Mortality caused by Wernicke's disease reaches 17% of diseases, which means 3.4/1000 or about 25 million contemporaries. The number of people with Wernicke's disease may be even higher, considering that early stages may have dysfunctions prior to the production of observable lesions at necropsy. In addition, uncounted numbers of people can experience fetal damage and subsequent diseases.

Pathophysiology

Thiamine in the human body has a half-life of 18 days and is quickly exhausted, particularly when metabolic demands exceed intake. A derivative of thiamine, thiamine pyrophosphate (TPP), is a cofactor involved in the citric acid cycle, as well as connecting the breakdown of sugars with the citric acid cycle. The citric acid cycle is a central metabolic pathway involved in the regulation of carbohydrate, lipid, and amino acid metabolism, and its disruption due to thiamine deficiency inhibits the production of many molecules including the neurotransmitters glutamic acid and GABA. Additionally thiamine may also be directly involved in neuromodulation.

Treatment

Many people with beriberi can be treated with thiamine alone. Given thiamine intravenously (and later orally), rapid and dramatic recovery can occur within hours. In situations where concentrated thiamine supplements are unavailable, feeding the person with a thiamine-rich diet (e.g. whole grain brown bread) will lead to recovery, though at a much slower rate.

Epidemiology

Historically beriberi was associated with a diet including much polished rice (white rice); when the relationship between polishing rice and the disease was discovered, it became possible to prevent and treat the deficiency condition, for example with inexpensive rice bran. Beriberi caused by inadequate nutritional intake is rare today in developed countries because of quality of food and the fact that many foods are fortified with vitamins. No reliable statistics are given for beriberi in developed countries in the 19th century or earlier; neither are statistics available before the last century in countries in extreme poverty.

Beriberi is a recurrent nutritional disease in detention houses even in this century. In 1999, an outbreak of beriberi occurred in a detention center in Taiwan. High rates of illness and death in overcrowded Haitian jails were traced in 2007 to the traditional practice of washing rice before cooking. In the Ivory Coast, among a group of prisoners with heavy punishment, 64% were affected by beriberi. Before beginning treatment, prisoners exhibited symptoms of dry or wet beriberi with neurological signs (swarming: 41%), cardiovascular signs (dyspnoea: 42%, thoracic pain: 35%), and oedemas of the lower limbs (51%). With treatment the rate of healing was about 97%.

Populations under extreme stress may be at higher risk for beriberi. Displaced populations, such as refugees from war, are susceptible to micronutritional deficiency, including beriberi. The severe nutritional deprivation caused by famine also can cause beriberis, although symptoms may be overlooked in clinical assessment or masked by other famine-related problems. An extreme weight-loss diet can, rarely, induce a famine-like state and the accompanying beriberi.

History

Etymology

According to the Oxford English Dictionary, the term 'beriberi' comes from a Sinhalese phrase meaning "weak, weak" or "I cannot, I cannot", the word being duplicated for emphasis.

According to Jacobus Bontius (Jacob de Bondt; 1591–1631), a Dutch physician who encountered the disease while working in Java in 1630, In the first known description of beriberi (or, *beri-beri*), he wrote: "A certain very troublesome affliction, which attacks men, is called by the inhabitants beriberi (which means sheep). I believe those, whom this same disease attacks, with their knees shaking and the legs raised up, walk like sheep. It is a kind of paralysis, or rather tremor: for it penetrates the motion and sensation of the hands and feet indeed sometimes of the whole body."

Identification

In the late 19th century, beriberi was studied by Takaki Kanehiro, a British-trained Japanese medical doctor of the Japanese Navy. Beriberi was a serious problem in the Japanese navy: sailors fell ill an average of four times a year in the period 1878 to 1881, and 35% were cases of beriberi. In 1883, Kanehiro learned of a very high incidence of beriberi among cadets on a training mission from Japan to Hawaii, via New Zealand and South America. The voyage lasted more than 9 months and resulted in 169 cases of sickness and 25 deaths on a ship of 376 men. With the support of the Japanese Navy, he conducted an experiment in which another ship was deployed on the same route, except that its crew was fed a diet of meat, fish, barley, rice, and beans. At the end of the voyage, this crew had only 14 cases of beriberi and no deaths. This convinced Kanehiro and the Japanese Navy that diet was the cause. In 1884, Kanehiro observed that beriberi was endemic among low-ranking crew who were often provided free rice and thus ate little else, but not among crews of Western navies and nor among Japanese officers who consumed a more varied diet.

In 1897, Christiaan Eijkman, a Dutch physician and pathologist, demonstrated that beriberi is caused by poor diet, and discovered that feeding unpolished rice (instead of the polished variety) to chickens helped to prevent beriberi. The following year, Sir Frederick Hopkins postulated that some foods contained "accessory factors"—in addition to proteins, carbohydrates, fats, and salt—that were necessary for the functions of the human body. In 1901, Gerrit Grijns (May 28, 1865 – November 11, 1944), a Dutch physician and assistant to Christiaan Eijkman in the Netherlands, correctly interpreted the disease as a deficiency syndrome, and between 1910 and 1913, Edward Bright Vedder established that an extract of rice bran is a treatment for beriberi. In 1929, Eijkman and Hopkins were awarded the Nobel Prize for Physiology or Medicine for their discoveries.

Stunted Growth

Stunted growth, also known as stunting and nutritional stunting, is a reduced growth rate in human development. It is a primary manifestation of malnutrition (or more precisely undernutrition) and recurrent infections, such as diarrhea and helminthiasis, in early childhood and even before birth, due to malnutrition during fetal development brought on by a malnourished mother. The definition of stunting according to the World Health Organisation (WHO) is for the "height for age" value to be less than two standard deviations of the WHO Child Growth Standards median.

As of 2012 an estimated 162 million children under 5 years of age, or 25%, were stunted in 2012. More than 90% of the world's stunted children live in Africa and Asia, where respectively 36% and 56% of children are affected. Once established, stunting and its effects typically become permanent. Stunted children may never regain the height lost as a result of stunting, and most children will never gain the corresponding body weight. Living in an environment where many people defecate in the open due to lack of sanitation, is an important cause of stunted growth in children, for example in India.

Health Effects

Stunted growth in children has the following public health impacts apart from the obvious impact of shorter stature of the person affected:

- greater risk for illness and premature death
- may result in delayed mental development and therefore poorer school performance and later on reduced productivity in the work force
- reduced cognitive capacity
- Women of shorter stature have a greater risk for complications during child birth due to their smaller pelvis, and are at risk of delivering a baby with low birth weight

- Stunted growth can even be passed on to the next generation (this is called the "intergenerational cycle of malnutrition")

The impact of stunting on child development has been established in multiple studies. If a child is stunted at age 2 they will have higher risk of poor cognitive and educational achievement in life, with subsequent socio-economic and inter-generational consequences. Multi-country studies have also suggested that stunting is associated with reductions in schooling, decreased economic productivity and poverty. Stunted children also display higher risk of developing chronic non-communicable conditions such as diabetes and obesity as adults. If a stunted child undergoes substantial weight gain after age 2, there is a higher chance of becoming obese. This is believed to be caused by metabolic changes produced by chronic malnutrition, that can produce metabolic imbalances if the individual is exposed to excessive or poor quality diets as an adult. This can lead to higher risk of developing other related non-communicable diseases such as hypertension, coronary heart disease, metabolic syndrome and stroke. At societal level, stunted individuals do not fulfill their physical and cognitive developmental potential and will not be able to contribute maximally to society. Stunting can therefore limit economic development and productivity, and it has been estimated that it can affect a country's GDP up to 3%.

Causes

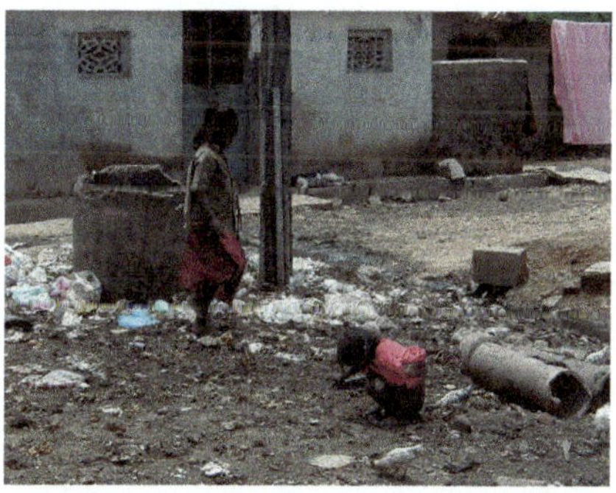

Children living in unsanitary conditions in an urban slum in India, at risk of diarrhea and stunted growth

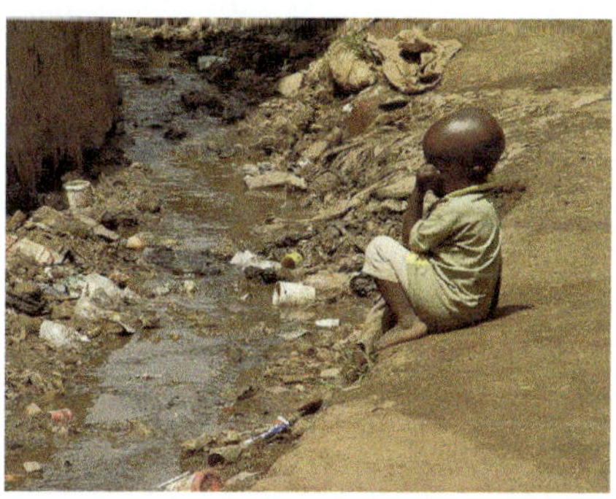

Child next to open sewer in slum in Kampala, Uganda, at risk of diarrhea and stunted growth

The causes for stunting are principally very similar if not the same as the causes for malnutrition in children. Most stunting happens during the 1,000-day period that spans from conception to a child's second birthday. The three main causes of stunting in South Asia, and probably in most developing countries, are poor feeding practices, poor maternal nutrition, and poor sanitation.

Feeding Practices

Inadequate complementary child feeding and a general lack of vital nutrients beside pure caloric intake is one cause for stunted growth. Children need to be fed diets which meet the minimum requirements in terms of frequency and diversity in order to prevent undernutrition.

Maternal Nutrition

Poor maternal nutrition during pregnancy and breastfeeding can lead to stunted growth of their children. Women who are underweight or anemic during pregnancy, are more likely to have stunted children which perpetuates the inter-generational transmission of stunting.

Sanitation

There is most likely a link between children's linear growth and household sanitation practices. The ingestion of high quantities of fecal bacteria by young children through putting soiled fingers or household items in the mouth leads to intestinal infections. This affect children's nutritional status by diminishing appetite, reducing nutrient absorption, and increasing nutrient losses.

The diseases recurrent diarrhoea and intestinal worm infections (helminthiasis) which are both linked to poor sanitation have been shown to contribute to child stunting. The evidence that a condition called environmental enteropathy also stunts children is not conclusively available yet, although the link is plausible and several studies are underway on this topic. Environmental enteropathy is a syndrome causing changes in the small intestine of persons and can be brought on due to lacking basic sanitary facilities and being exposed to faecal contamination on a long-term basis.

Research on a global level has found that the proportion of stunting that could be attributed to five or more episodes of diarrhoea before two years of age was 25%. Since diarrhoea is closely linked with water, sanitation and hygiene (WASH), this is a good indicator for the connection between WASH and stunted growth. To what extent improvements in drinking water safety, toilet use and good handwashing practices contribute to reduce stunting depends on the how bad these practices were prior to interventions.

Diagnosis

Growth stunting is identified by comparing measurements of children's heights to the World Health Organization 2006 growth reference population: children who fall below the fifth percentile of the reference population in height for age are defined as stunted, regardless of the reason. The lower than fifth percentile corresponds to less than two standard deviations of the WHO Child Growth Standards median.

As an indicator of nutritional status, comparisons of children's measurements with growth reference curves may be used differently for populations of children than for individual children. The fact that an individual child falls below the fifth percentile for height for age on a growth reference curve may reflect normal variation in growth within a population: the individual child may be short simply because both parents carried genes for shortness and not because of inadequate nutrition. However, if substantially more than 5% of an identified child population have height for age that is less than the fifth percentile on the reference curve, then the population is said to have a higher-than-expected prevalence of stunting, and malnutrition is generally the first cause considered.

Prevention

Three main things are needed to reduce stunting:

- a kind of environment where political commitment can thrive (also called an "enabling environment")
- applying several nutritional modifications or changes in a population on a large scale which have a high benefit and a low cost
- a strong foundation that can drive change (food security, empowerment of women and a supportive health environment through increasing access to safe water and sanitation).

To prevent stunting, it is not just a matter of providing better nutrition but also access to clean water, improved sanitation (hygienic toilets) and hand washing at critical times (summarised as "WASH"). Without provision of toilets, prevention of tropical intestinal diseases, which may affect almost all children in the developing world and lead to stunting will not be possible.

Studies have looked at ranking the underlying determinants in terms of their potency in reducing child stunting and found in the order of potency:

- percent of dietary energy from non-staples (greatest impact)
- access to sanitation and women's education
- access to safe water
- women's empowerment as measured by the female-to-male life expectancy ratio
- per capita dietary energy supply

Three of these determinants should receive attention in particular: access to sanitation, diversity of calorie sources from food supplies, and women's empowerment. A study by the Institute of Development Studies has stressed that: "The first two should be prioritized because they have strong impacts yet are farthest below their desired levels".

The goal of UN agencies, governments and NGO is now to optimise nutrition during the first 1000 days of a child's life, from pregnancy to the child's second birthday, in order to reduce the prevalence of stunting. The first 1000 days in a child's life are a crucial "window of opportunity" because the brain develops rapidly, laying the foundation for future cognitive and social ability. Furthermore, it is also the time when young children are the most at risk of infections that lead to diarrhoea. It is the time when they stop breast feeding (weaning process), begin to crawl, put things in their mouths and become exposed to faecal matter from open defecation and environmental enteropathies.

Pregnant and Lactating Mothers

Ensuring proper nutrition of pregnant and lactating mothers is essential. Achieving so by helping women of reproductive age be in good nutritional status at conception is an excellent preventive measure. A focus on the pre-conception period has recently been introduced as a complement to the key phase of the 1000 days of pregnancy and first two years of life. An example of this is are attempts to control anemia in women of reproductive age. A well-nourished mother is the first step of stunting prevention, decreasing chances of the baby being born of low birth-weight, which is the first risk factor for future malnutrition.

After birth, in terms of interventions for the child, early initiation of breastfeeding, together with exclusive breastfeeding for the first 6 months, are pillars of stunting prevention. Introducing proper complementary feeding after 6 months of age together with breastfeeding until age 2 is the next step.

Policy Interventions

In summary, key policy interventions for the prevention of stunting are:

- Improvement in nutrition surveillance activities to identify rates and trends of stunting and other forms of malnutrition within countries. This should be done with an equity perspective, as it is likely that stunting rates will vary greatly between different population groups. The most vulnerable should be prioritized. The same should be done for risk factors such as anemia, maternal under-nutrition, food insecurity, low birth-weight, breastfeeding practices etc. By collecting more detailed information, it is easier to ensure that policy interventions really address the root causes of stunting.
- Political will to develop and implement national targets and strategies in line with evidence-based international guidelines as well as contextual factors.

- Designing and implementing policies promoting nutritional and health well-being of mothers and women of reproductive age. The main focus should be on the 1000 days of pregnancy and first two years of life, but the pre-conception period should not be neglected as it can play a significant role in ensuring the fetus and baby's nutrition.
- Designing and implementing policies promoting proper breastfeeding and complementary feeding practice (focusing on diet diversity for both macro and micronutrients). This can ensure optimal infant nutrition as well as protection from infections that can weaken the child's body. Labor policy ensuring mothers have the chance to breastfeed should be considered where necessary.
- Introducing interventions addressing social and other health determinants of stunting, such as poor sanitation and access to drinking water, early marriages, intestinal parasite infections, malaria and other childhood preventable disease (referred to as "nutrition-sensitive interventions"), as well as the country's food security landscape. Interventions to keep adolescent girls in school can be effective at delaying marriage with subsequent nutritional benefits for both women and babies. Regulating milk substitutes is also very important to ensure that as many mothers as possible breastfeed their babies, unless a clear contraindication is present.
- Broadly speaking, effective policies to reduce stunting require multisectoral approaches, strong political commitment, community involvement and integrated service delivery.

Epidemiology

According to the World Health organisation if less than 20% of the population is affected by stunting, this is regarded as "low prevalence" in terms of public health significance. Values of 40% or more are regarded as very high prevalence, and values in between as medium to high prevalence.

UNICEF has estimated that: "Globally, more than one quarter (26 per cent) of children under 5 years of age were stunted in 2011 – roughly 165 million children worldwide." and "In sub-Saharan Africa, 40 per cent of children under 5 years of age are stunted; in South Asia, 39 per cent are stunted." The four countries with the highest prevalence are Timor-Leste, Burundi, Niger and Madagascar where more than half of children under 5 years old are stunted.

Trends

As of 2015, it was estimated that there were 156 million stunted children under 5 in the world, 90% of them living in low and low-middle income countries. 56% of these were in Asia, and 37% in Africa. It is possible that some of these children concurrently had other forms of malnutrition, including wasting and stunting, and overweight and stunting. No statistics are currently available for these combined conditions. Stunting has been on the decline for the past 15 years, but this decline has been too slow. As a comparison, there were 255 million stunted children in 1990, 224 in 1995, 198 in 2000, 182 in 2005, 169 in 2010, and 156 in 2016. The decline is happening, but it is uneven geographically, it is unequal among different groups in society, and prevalence of stunting remains at unacceptably high numbers. Too many children who are not able to fulfill their genetic physical and cognitive developmental potential.

Over the period 2000-2015, Asia reduced its stunting prevalence from 38 to 24%, Africa from 38 to 32%, and Latin America and the Caribbean from 18 to 11%. This equates to a relative reduction of 36, 17 and 39% respectively, indicating that Asia and Latin America and the Caribbean have displayed much larger improvements than Africa, which needs to address this issue with much more effort if it is to win the battle against a problem that has been crippling its development for decades. Of these regions, Latin America and the Caribbean are on track to achieve global targets set with global initiatives such as the United Nations Millennium Development Goals and the World Health Assembly targets.

Sub-regional stunting rates are as follows: In Africa, the highest rates are observed in East Africa (37.5%). All other Sub-Saharan sub-regions also have high rates, with 32.1% in West Africa, 31.2% in Central Africa, and 28.4% in Southern Africa. North Africa is at 18%, and the Middle East at 16.2%. In Asia, the highest rate is observed in South Asia at 34.4%. South-East Asia is at 26.3%. Pacific Islands also display a high rate at 38.2%. Central and South America are respectively at 15.6 and 9.9%. South Asia, given its very high population at over 1 billion and high prevalence rate of stunting, is the region currently hosting the highest absolute number of children with stunting (60 million plus).

Looking at absolute numbers of children under 5 affected by stunting, it is obvious why current efforts and reductions are insufficient. The absolute number of stunted children has increased in Africa from 50.4 to 58.5 million in the time 2000-2015. This is despite the reduction in percentage prevalence of stunting, and is due to the high rates of population growth. The data therefore indicate that the rate of reduction of stunting in Africa has not been able to counterbalance the increased number of growing children that fall into the trap of malnutrition, due to population growth in the region. This is also true in Oceania, unlike Asia and Latin America and the Caribbean where substantial absolute reductions in the number of stunted children have been observed (for example, Asia reduced its number of stunted children from 133 million to 88 million between 2000 and 2015).

The reduction in stunting is closely linked to poverty reduction and the will and ability of governments to set up solid multisectoral approaches to reduce chronic malnutrition. Low income countries are the only group with more stunted children today than in the year 2000. Conversely, all other countries (high-income, upper-middle income, lower-middle income) have achieved reductions in the numbers of stunted children. This sadly perpetuates a vicious cycle of poverty and malnutrition, whereby malnourished children are not able to maximally contribute to economic development as adults, and poverty increases chances of malnutrition.

Research

The Water and Sanitation Program of the World Bank has investigated links between lack of sanitation and stunting in Vietnam and Lao PDR. For example, in Vietnam it was found that lack of sanitation in rural villages in mountainous regions of Vietnam led to five-year-old children being 3.7 cm shorter than healthy children living in villages with good access to sanitation. This difference in height is irreversible and matters a great deal for a child's cognitive development and future productive potential.

Review Articles

The Lancet has published two comprehensive series on maternal and child nutrition, in 2008 and 2013. The series review the epidemiology of global malnutrition and analyze the state of the evidence for cost-effective interventions that should be scaled-up to achieve impact and global targets. In the first of such series, investigators define the importance of the 1000 day and identify child malnutrition as being responsible for one third of all child deaths worldwide. This finding is key in that it points at malnutrition as a key determinant of child mortality that is often overlooked. When a child dies of pneumonia, malaria or diarrhea (some of the causes of child mortality in the world), it may well be that malnutrition is a key contributing factor that prevents the body from successfully fighting the infection and recovering from the disease. In the follow up series in 2013, the focus on undernutrition is expanded to the increasing burden of obesity in both high, middle and low income countries. Interestingly, several countries with high levels of child stunting and undernutrition are starting to display worrisome increasing trends of child obesity concurrently, due to increased wealth and the persistence of significant inequalities. The challenges these countries face are particularly difficult as they require intervening on two levels on what has come to be called "double burden of malnutrition". As an example, in India 30% of children under 5 years of age are stunted, and 20% are overweight. Neglecting these nutritional problems is not an option anymore if countries are to escape poverty traps and provide opportunities to their people to live fulfilling productive lives without stunting.

Examples

The 2012 World Health Assembly, with its 194 member states, convened to discuss global issues of maternal, infant and young child nutrition, and developed a plan with 6 targets for 2025. The first of such targets aims to reduce by 40% the number of children who are stunted in the world, by 2025. This would correspond to 100 million stunted children in 2025. At the current reduction rate, the predicted number in 2025 will be

127 million, indicating the need to scale-up and intensify efforts if the global community is to reach its goals.

The World Bank estimates that the extra cost to achieve the reduction goal will be $8.50 yearly per stunted child, for a total of $49.6 Billion for the next decade. Stunting has been shown to be one of the most cost-effective global health problems to invest in, with an estimated return on investment of $18 for every dollar spent thanks to its impact on economic productivity. Despite the evidence in favor of investing in the reduction of stunting, current investments are too low at about $2.9 billion per year, with $1.6 billion coming from Governments, $0.2 billion from donors, and $1.1 paid by individuals.

Sustainable Development Goals

In 2015, the United Nations and its member states agreed on a new sustainable development agenda to promote prosperity and reduce poverty, putting forward 17 Sustainable Development Goals (SDGs) to be achieved by 2030. SDG 2 aims to "End hunger, achieve food security and improved nutrition, and promote sustainable agriculture". Sub-goal 2.2. aims to "by 2030 end all forms of malnutrition, including achieving by 2025 the internationally agreed targets on stunting and wasting in children under five years of age, and address the nutritional needs of adolescent girls, pregnant and lactating women, and older persons".

The global community has recognized more and more the critical importance of stunting during the past decade. Investments to address it have increased but remain far from being sufficient to solve it and unleash the human potential that remains trapped in malnutrition.

The "Scaling Up Nutrition Movement (SUN)" movement is the main network of governments, non-governmental and international organizations, donors, private companies and academic institutions working together in pursuit of improved global nutrition and a world without hunger and malnutrition. It was launched at the UN General Assembly of 2010 and it calls for country-led multi-sectoral strategies to address child malnutrition by scaling-up evidence-based interventions in both nutrition specific and sensitive areas. As of 2016, 50 countries have joined the SUN Movement with strategies that are aligned with international frameworks of action.

Brazil

Brazil displayed a remarkable reduction in the rates of child stunting under age 5, from 37% in 1974, to 7.1% in 2007. This happened in association with impressive social and economic development that reduced the numbers of Brazilians living in extreme poverty (less than $1.25 per day) from 25.6% in 1990 to 4.8% in 2008. The successful reduction in child malnutrition in Brazil can be attributed to strong political commitment that led to improvements in the water and sanitation system, increased female schooling, scale-up of quality maternal and child health services, increased economic power at family level (including successful cash transfer programs), and improvements in food security throughout the country.

Peru

After a decade (1995-2005) in which stunting rates stagnated in the country, Peru designed and implemented a national strategy against child malnutrition called crecer ("grow"), which complemented a social development conditional cash-transfer program called juntos, which included a nutritional component. The strategy was multisectoral in that it involved the health, education, water, sanitation and hygiene, agriculture and housing sectors and stakeholders. It was led by the Government and the Prime Minister himself, and included non-governmental partners at both central, regional and community level. After the strategy was implemented, stunting went from 22.9% to 17.9% (2005-2010), with very significant improvements in rural areas where it had been more difficult to reduce stunting rates in the past.

India (Maharashtra)

The State of Maharashtra in Central-Western India has been able to produce an impressive reduction in stunting rates in children under 2 years of age from 44% to 22.8% in the 2005-2012 period. This is particularly remarkable given the immense challenges India has faced to address malnutrition, and that the Country host almost half of all stunted children under 5 in the world. This was achieved through integrated community-based programs that were designed by a central advisory body that promoted multisectoral collaboration, provided advice to policy-makers on evidence-based solutions, and advocated for the key role of the 1000 days (pregnancy and first two years of life).

Wasting

In medicine, wasting, also known as wasting syndrome, refers to the process by which a debilitating disease causes muscle and fat tissue to "waste" away. Wasting is sometimes referred to as "acute malnutrition" because it is believed that episodes of wasting have a short duration, in contrast to stunting, which is regarded as chronic malnutrition. According to the latest UN estimates, an estimated 52 million children under 5 years of age, or 8%, were wasted in 2011. The vast majority, about 70%, of the world's wasted children live in Asia, most in South-Central Asia.

Causes

Wasting can be caused by an extremely low energy intake (e.g., caused by famine), nutrient losses due to infection, or a combination of low intake and high loss. Infections and conditions associated with wasting include tuberculosis, chronic diarrhea, AIDS, and superior mesenteric artery syndrome. The mechanism may involve cachectin – also called tumor necrosis factor, a macrophage-secreted cytokine. Caretakers and health providers can sometimes contribute to wasting if the patient is placed on an improper diet. Voluntary weight loss and eating disorders are excluded as causes of wasting.

Classification

- Children: Weight-for-height (WFH). In infants under 24 months, recumbent (supine) length is used. WFH as % of median reference value is calculated this way:

$$\text{WFH} = \frac{\text{weight of a given child}}{\text{median weight for a given child of that height}} \times 100$$

Cutoff points may vary, but <80% (close to −2 Z-score) is often used.

- Adults:
  - o Body Mass Index (BMI) is the quotient between weight and height squared (kg/m^2). An individual with a BMI < 18.5 is regarded as a case of wasting.
  - o Percent of body weight lost (At Tufts, an unintentional loss of 6% or more in 6 months is regarded as wasting)

Treatment

Antiretrovirals and anabolic steroids have been used to treat HIV wasting syndrome. Additionally, an increase in protein-rich foods such as peanut butter, eggs, and cheese can assist in controlling the loss of muscle mass.

Scurvy

Scurvy is a disease resulting from a lack of vitamin C. Early symptoms include weakness, feeling tired, curly hair, and sore arms and legs. Without treatment, decreased red blood cells, gum disease, and bleeding from the skin may occur. As scurvy worsens there can be poor wound healing, personality changes, and finally death from infection or bleeding.

Scurvy is caused by not enough vitamin C in the diet. It typically takes at least a month of little to no vitamin C before symptoms occur. In modern times, it occurs most commonly in people with mental disorders, unusual eating habits, alcoholism, and old people who live alone. Other risk factors include intestinal malabsorption and dialysis. Humans and certain other animals require vitamin C in their diets to make the building blocks for collagen. Diagnosis is typically based on physical signs, X-rays, and improvement after treatment.

Treatment is with vitamin C supplements taken by mouth. Improvement often begins in a few days with complete recovery in a few weeks. Sources of vitamin C in the diet include citrus fruit and a number of vegetables such as tomatoes and potatoes. Cooking often decreases vitamin C in foods.

Scurvy is currently rare. It occurs more often in the developing world in association with malnutrition. Rates among refugees are reported at 5% to 45%. Scurvy was described as early as the time of ancient Egypt. It was a limiting factor in long distance sea travel, often killing large numbers of people. A Scottish surgeon in the Royal Navy, James Lind, was the first to prove it could be treated with citrus fruit in a 1753 publication. His experiments represented the first controlled trial. It took another 40 years before the British Navy began giving out lemon juice routinely.

Signs and Symptoms

Early symptoms are malaise and lethargy. Even earlier might be a pain in a section of the gums which interferes with digestion. After 1–3 months, patients develop shortness of breath and bone pain. Myalgias may occur because of reduced carnitine production. Other symptoms include skin changes with roughness, easy bruising and petechiae, gum disease, loosening of teeth, poor wound healing, and emotional changes (which may appear before any physical changes). Dry mouth and dry eyes similar to Sjögren's syndrome may occur. In the late stages, jaundice, generalized edema, oliguria, neuropathy, fever, convulsions, and eventual death are frequently seen.

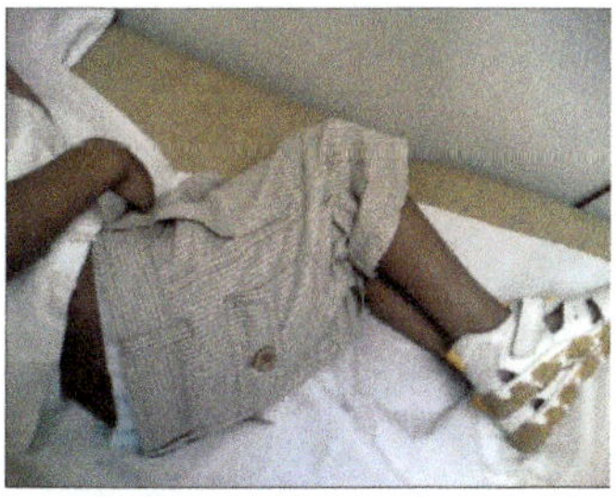

A child with scurvy in flexion posture.

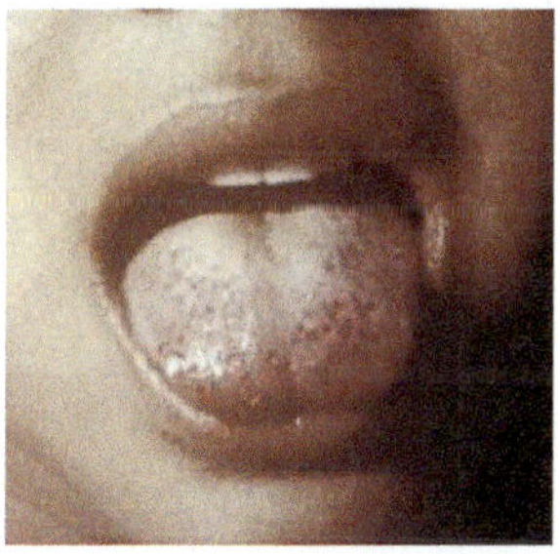

A child presenting a "scorbutic tongue" due to what proved to be a vitamin C deficiency.

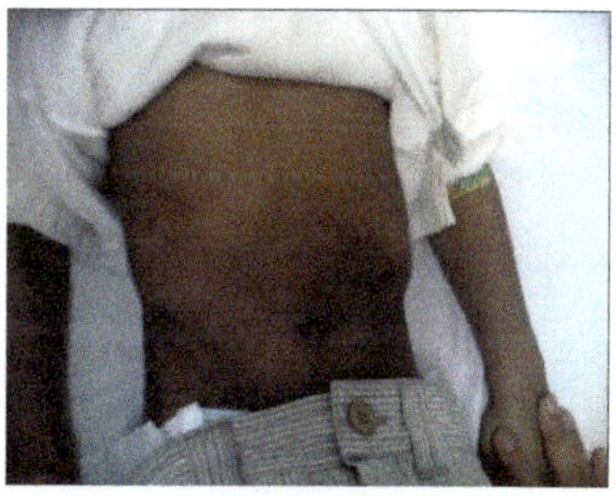

Photo of the chest cage with pectus excavatum and scorbutic rosaries.

Cause

Scurvy or subclinical scurvy is caused by the lack of vitamin C. In modern Western societies, scurvy is rarely present in adults, although infants and elderly people are affected.

Virtually all commercially available baby formulas contain added vitamin C. Human breast milk contains sufficient vitamin C, if the mother has an adequate intake.

Scurvy is one of the accompanying diseases of malnutrition (other such micronutrient deficiencies are beriberi or pellagra) and thus is still widespread in areas of the world depending on external food aid. Though rare, there are also documented cases of scurvy due to poor dietary choices by people living in industrialized nations.

Pathogenesis

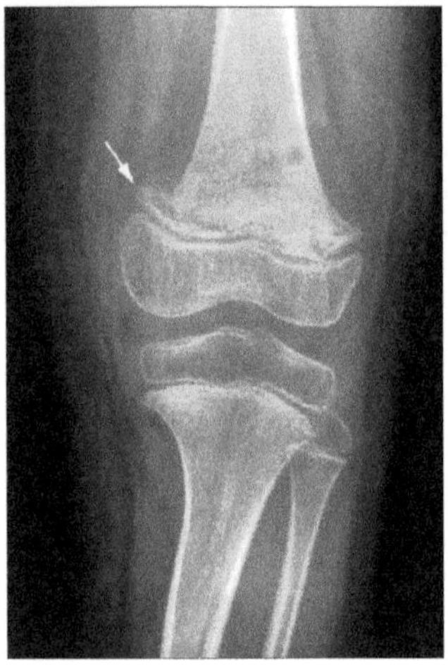

X-ray of the knee joint (arrow indicates scurvy line).

Ascorbic acid is needed for a variety of biosynthetic pathways, by accelerating hydroxylation and amidation reactions. In the synthesis of collagen, ascorbic acid is required as a cofactor for prolyl hydroxylase and lysyl hydroxylase. These two enzymes are responsible for the hydroxylation of the proline and lysine amino acids in collagen. Hydroxyproline and hydroxylysine are important for stabilizing collagen by cross-linking the propeptides in collagen. Defective collagen fibrillogenesis impairs wound healing. Collagen is an important part of bone, so bone formation is affected. Defective connective tissue leads to fragile capillaries, resulting in abnormal bleeding. Untreated scurvy is invariably fatal.

Prevention

Scurvy can be prevented by a diet that includes vitamin C-rich foods such as bell peppers (sweet peppers), blackcurrants, broccoli, guava, kiwifruit, and parsley. Other sources rich in vitamin C are fruits such as lemons, oranges, papaya, and strawberries. It is also found in vegetables, such as brussels sprouts, cabbage, potatoes, and spinach. Some fruits and vegetables not high in vitamin C may be pickled in lemon juice, which is high in vitamin C. Though redundant in the presence of a balanced diet, various nutritional supplements are available that provide ascorbic acid well in excess of that required to prevent scurvy.

Some animal products, including liver, Muktuk (whale skin), oysters, and parts of the central nervous system, including the adrenal medulla, brain, and spinal cord, contain large amounts of vitamin C, and can even be used to treat scurvy. Fresh meat from animals which make their own vitamin C (which most animals do) contains enough vitamin C to prevent scurvy, and even partly treat it. In some cases (notably French soldiers eating fresh horse meat), it was discovered that meat alone, even partly cooked meat, could alleviate scurvy. Conversely, in other cases, a meat-only diet could cause scurvy.

Scott's 1902 Antarctic expedition used lightly fried seal meat and liver, whereby complete recovery from incipient scurvy was reported to have taken less than two weeks.

History

Hippocrates documented scurvy as a disease, and Egyptians have recorded its symptoms as early as 1550 BCE. The knowledge that consuming foods containing vitamin C is a cure for scurvy has been repeatedly rediscovered and forgotten into the early 20th century.

Early Modern Era

In the 13th century, the Crusaders frequently suffered from scurvy. In the 1497 expedition of Vasco de Gama, the curative effects of citrus fruit were already known and confirmed by Pedro Álvares Cabral and his crew in 1507.

The Portuguese planted fruit trees and vegetables in Saint Helena, a stopping point for homebound voyages from Asia, and left their sick, suffering from scurvy and other ailments, to be taken home, if they recovered, by the next ship.

In 1500, one of the pilots of Cabral's fleet bound for India noted that in Malindi, its king offered the expedition fresh supplies such as lambs, chickens, and ducks, along with lemons and oranges, due to which "some of our ill were cured of scurvy".

Unfortunately, these travel accounts have not stopped further maritime tragedies caused by scurvy, first because of the lack of communication between travelers and those responsible for their health, and because fruits and vegetables could not be kept for long on ships.

In 1536, the French explorer Jacques Cartier, exploring the St. Lawrence River, used the local natives' knowledge to save his men who were dying of scurvy. He boiled the needles of the arbor vitae tree (Eastern White Cedar) to make a tea that was later shown to contain 50 mg of vitamin C per 100 grams. Such treatments were not available aboard ship, where the disease was most common.

During the Age of Exploration (between 1500 and 1800), it has been estimated that scurvy killed at least two million sailors. Jonathan Lamb wrote: "In 1499, Vasco da Gama lost 116 of his crew of 170; In 1520, Magellan lost 208 out of 230;...all mainly to scurvy."

In 1593, Admiral Sir Richard Hawkins advocated drinking orange and lemon juice as a means of preventing scurvy.

In 1614, John Woodall, Surgeon General of the East India Company, published "The Surgion's Mate" as a handbook for apprentice surgeons aboard the company's ships. He repeated the experience of mariners that the cure for scurvy was fresh food or, if not available, oranges, lemons, limes, and tamarinds. He was, however, unable to explain the reason why, and his assertion had no impact on the opinions of the influential physicians who ran the medical establishment that scurvy was a digestive complaint.

18th Century

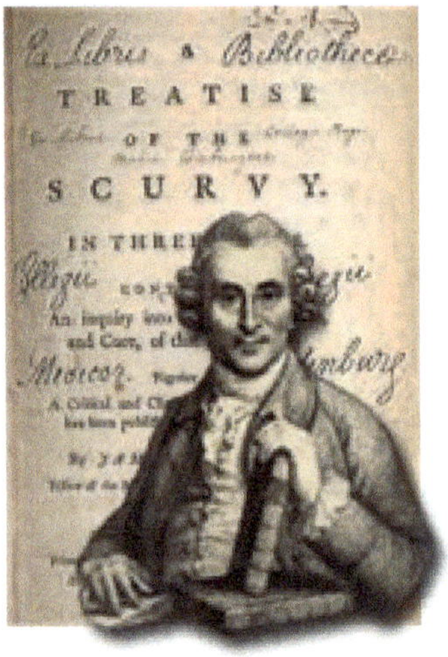

James Lind, a pioneer in the field of scurvy prevention

A 1707 handwritten book by Mrs. Ebot Mitchell, discovered in a house in Hasfield, Gloucestershire, contains a "Recp.t for the Scurvy" that consisted of extracts from various plants mixed with a plentiful supply of orange juice, white wine or beer.

In 1734, the Leiden-based physician Johann Bachstrom published a book on scurvy in which he stated, "scurvy is solely owing to a total abstinence from fresh vegetable food, and greens; which is alone the primary cause of the disease", and urged the use of fresh fruit and vegetables as a cure.

However, it was not until 1747 that James Lind formally demonstrated that scurvy could be treated by supplementing the diet with citrus fruit, in the first ever clinical trial. In 1753, Lind published *A Treatise of the Scurvy*, in which he explained the details of his clinical trial, but it occupied only a few paragraphs in a work that was long and complex and had little impact. In fact, Lind himself never actively promoted lemon juice as a single 'cure'. He shared medical opinion at the time that scurvy had multiple causes – notably hard work, bad water, and the consumption of salt meat in a damp atmosphere which inhibited healthful perspiration and normal excretion - and therefore required multiple solutions. He was also sidetracked by the possibilities of producing a concentrated 'rob' of lemon juice by boiling it. Unfortunately this process destroyed the vitamin C and was unsuccessful.

During the 18th century, disease killed more British sailors than enemy action. It was mainly by scurvy that George Anson, in his celebrated voyage of 1740–1744, lost nearly two-thirds of his crew (1300 out of 2000) within the first 10 months of the voyage. The Royal Navy enlisted 184,899 sailors during the Seven Years' War; 133,708 of these were "missing" or died from disease, and scurvy was the leading cause.

Although throughout this period sailors and naval surgeons were increasingly convinced that citrus fruits could cure scurvy, the classically trained physicians who ran the medical establishment dismissed this evidence as mere anecdote which did not conform to current theories of disease. Literature championing the cause of citrus juice, therefore, had no practical impact. Medical theory was based on the assumption that scurvy was a disease of internal putrefaction brought on by faulty digestion caused by the hardships of life at sea and the naval diet. Although this basic idea was given different emphases by successive theorists, the remedies they advocated (and which the navy accepted) amounted to little more than the consumption of 'fizzy drinks' to activate the digestive system, the most extreme of which was the regular consumption of 'elixir of vitriol' – sulphuric acid taken with spirits and barley water, and laced with spices.

In 1764, a new variant appeared. Advocated by Dr David McBride and Sir John Pringle, Surgeon General of the Army and later President of the Royal Society, this idea was that scurvy was the result of a lack of 'fixed air' in the tissues which could be prevented by drinking infusions of malt and wort whose fermentation within the body would stimulate digestion and restore the missing gases. These ideas received wide and influential backing, when James Cook set off to circumnavigate the world (1768–1771) in HM Bark *Endeavour*, malt and wort were top of the list of the remedies he was ordered to investigate. The others were beer, sour crout and Lind's 'rob'. The list did not include lemons.

Cook did not lose a single man to scurvy, and his report came down in favour of malt and wort, although it is now clear that the reason for the health of his crews on this and other voyages was Cook's regime of shipboard cleanliness, enforced by strict discipline, as well as frequent replenishment of fresh food and green stuffs. Another rule implemented by Cook was his prohibition of the consumption of salt fat skimmed from the ship's copper boiling pans, then a common practice in the Navy. In contact with air the copper formed compounds that prevented the absorption of vitamins by the intestines.

The first major long distance expedition that experienced virtually no scurvy was that of the Spanish naval officer Alessandro Malaspina, 1789–1794. Malaspina's medical officer, Pedro González, was convinced that fresh oranges and lemons were essential for preventing scurvy. Only one outbreak occurred, during a 56-day trip across the open sea. Five sailors came down with symptoms, one seriously. After three days at Guam all five were healthy again. Spain's large empire and many ports of call made it easier to acquire fresh fruit.

Although towards the end of the century MacBride's theories were being challenged, the medical establishment in Britain remained wedded to the notion that scurvy was a disease of internal 'putrefaction' and the Sick and Hurt Board, run by administrators, felt obliged to follow its advice. Within the Royal Navy, however, opinion - strengthened by first-hand experience of the use of lemon juice at the siege of Gibraltar and during Admiral Rodney's expedition to the Caribbean - had become increasingly convinced of its efficacy. This was reinforced by the writings of experts like Gilbert Blane and Thomas Trotter and by the reports of up-and-coming naval commanders.

With the coming of war in 1793, the need to eliminate scurvy acquired a new urgency. But the first initiative came not from the medical establishment but from the admirals. Ordered to lead an expedition against Mauritius, Rear Admiral Gardner was uninterested in the wort, malt and elixir of vitriol which were still being issued to ships of the Royal Navy, and demanded that he be supplied with lemons, to counteract scurvy on the voyage. Members of the Sick and Hurt Board, recently augmented by two practical naval surgeons, supported the request, and the Admiralty ordered that it be done. There was, however, a last minute change of plan. The expedition against Mauritius was cancelled. On 2 May 1794, only HMS *Suffolk* and two sloops under Commodore Peter Rainier sailed for the east with an outward bound convoy, but the warships were fully supplied with lemon juice and the sugar with which it had to be mixed. Then in March 1795, came astonishing news. *Suffolk* had arrived in India after a four-month voyage without a trace of scurvy and with a crew that was healthier than when it set out.

The effect was immediate. Fleet commanders clamoured also to be supplied with lemon juice, and by June the Admiralty acknowledged the groundswell of demand in the navy had agreed to a proposal from the Sick and Hurt Board that lemon juice and sugar should in future be issued as a daily ration to the crews of all warships.

It took a few years before the method of distribution to all ships in the fleet had been perfected and the supply of the huge quantities of lemon juice required to be secured, but by 1800, the system was in place and functioning. This led to a remarkable health improvement among the sailors and consequently played a critical role in gaining the advantage in naval battles against enemies who had yet to introduce the measures.

19th Century

The surgeon-in-chief of Napoleon's army at the Siege of Alexandria (1801), Baron Dominique-Jean Larrey, wrote in his memoirs that the consumption of horse meat helped the French to curb an epidemic of scurvy. The meat was cooked but was freshly obtained from young horses bought from Arabs, and was nevertheless effective. This helped to start the 19th-century tradition of horse meat consumption in France.

Lauchlin Rose patented a method used to preserve citrus juice without alcohol in 1867, creating a concentrated drink known as Rose's lime juice. The Merchant Shipping Act of 1867 required all ships of the Royal Navy and Merchant Navy to provide a daily lime ration to sailors to prevent scurvy. The product became nearly ubiquitous, hence the term "limey", first for British sailors, then for English immigrants within the former British colonies (particularly America, New Zealand and South Africa), and finally, in old American slang, all British people.

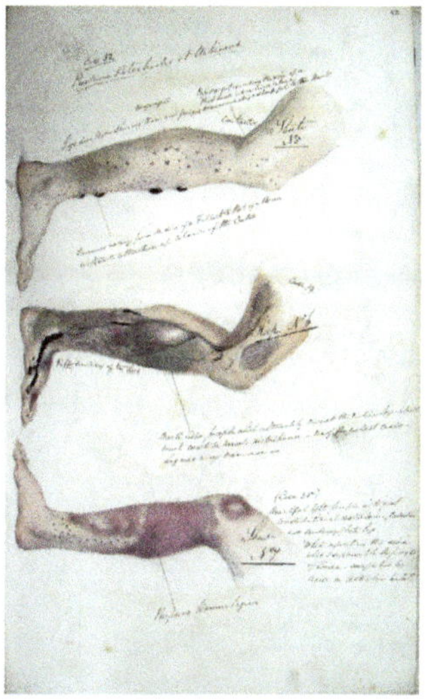

Page from the journal of Henry Walsh Mahon showing the effects of scurvy, from his time aboard HM Convict Ship *Barrosa* (1841/2)

The plant *Cochlearia officinalis*, also known as "Common Scurvygrass", acquired its common name from the observation that it cured scurvy, and it was taken on board ships in dried bundles or distilled extracts. Its very bitter taste was usually disguised with herbs and spices; however, this did not prevent scurvygrass drinks and sandwiches from becoming a popular fad in the UK until the middle of the nineteenth century, when citrus fruits became more readily available.

West Indian limes began to supplement lemons, when Spain's alliance with France against Britain in the Napoleonic Wars made the supply of Mediterranean lemons problematic, and because they were more easily obtained from Britain's Caribbean colonies and were believed to be more effective because they were more acidic. It was the acid, not the (then-unknown) Vitamin C that was believed to cure scurvy. In fact, the West Indian limes were significantly lower in Vitamin C than the previous lemons and further were not served fresh but rather as lime juice, which had been exposed to light and air, and piped through copper tubing, all of which significantly reduced the Vitamin C. Indeed, a 1918 animal experiment using representative samples of the Navy and Merchant Marine's lime juice showed that it had virtually no antiscorbutic power at all.

The belief that scurvy was fundamentally a nutritional deficiency, best treated by consumption of fresh food, particularly fresh citrus or fresh meat, was not universal in the 19th and early 20th centuries, and thus sailors and explorers continued to suffer from scurvy into the 20th century. For example, the Belgian Antarctic Expedition of

1897–1899 became seriously affected by scurvy when its leader, Adrien de Gerlache, initially discouraged his men from eating penguin and seal meat.

In the Royal Navy's Arctic expeditions in the 19th century it was widely believed that scurvy was prevented by good hygiene on board ship, regular exercise, and maintaining the morale of the crew, rather than by a diet of fresh food. Navy expeditions continued to be plagued by scurvy even while fresh (not jerked or tinned) meat was well known as a practical antiscorbutic among civilian whalers and explorers in the Arctic. Even cooking fresh meat did not entirely destroy its antiscorbutic properties, especially as many cooking methods failed to bring all the meat to high temperature.

The confusion is attributed to a number of factors:

- while *fresh* citrus (particularly lemons) cured scurvy, lime *juice* that had been exposed to light, air and copper tubing did not – thus undermining the theory that citrus cured scurvy;
- fresh meat (especially organ meat and raw meat, consumed in arctic exploration) also cured scurvy, undermining the theory that fresh vegetable matter was essential to preventing and curing scurvy;
- increased marine speed via steam shipping, and improved nutrition on land, reduced the incidence of scurvy – and thus the ineffectiveness of copper-piped lime juice compared to fresh lemons was not immediately revealed.

In the resulting confusion, a new hypothesis was proposed, following the new germ theory of disease – that scurvy was caused by ptomaine, a waste product of bacteria, particularly in tainted tinned meat.

Infantile scurvy emerged in the late 19th century because children were being fed pasteurized cow's milk, particularly in the urban upper class. While pasteurization killed bacteria, it also destroyed vitamin C. This was eventually resolved by supplementing with onion juice or cooked potatoes.

20th Century

By the early 20th century, when Robert Falcon Scott made his first expedition to the Antarctic (1901–1904), the prevailing theory was that scurvy was caused by "ptomaine poisoning", particularly in tinned meat. However, Scott discovered that a diet of fresh meat from Antarctic seals cured scurvy before any fatalities occurred.

In 1907, an animal model which would eventually help to isolate and identify the "antiscorbutic factor" was discovered. Axel Holst and Theodor Frølich, two Norwegian physicians studying shipboard beriberi contracted by ship's crews in the Norwegian Fishing Fleet, wanted a small test mammal to substitute for the pigeons then used in beriberi research. They fed guinea pigs their test diet of grains and flour, which had earlier produced beriberi in their pigeons, and were surprised when classic scurvy resulted instead. This was a serendipitous choice of animal. Until that time, scurvy had not been observed in any organism apart from humans and had been considered an exclusively human disease. (Some birds are susceptible to scurvy, but pigeons are unaffected by scurvy, as they produce vitamin C.) Holst and Frølich found they could cure scurvy in guinea pigs with the addition of various fresh foods and extracts. This discovery of an animal experimental model for scurvy, which was made even before the essential idea of "vitamins" in foods had been put forward, has been called the single most important piece of vitamin C research.

Vilhjalmur Stefansson, an arctic explorer who had lived among the Inuit, proved that the all-meat diet they consumed did not lead to vitamin deficiencies. He participated in a study in New York's Bellevue Hospital in February 1928, where he and a companion ate only meat for a year while under close medical observation, yet remained in good health.

In 1927, Hungarian biochemist Szent-Györgyi isolated a compound he called "hexuronic acid". Szent-Györgyi suspected hexuronic acid, which he had isolated from adrenal glands, to be the antiscorbutic agent, but he could not prove it without an animal-deficiency model. In 1932, the connection between hexuronic acid and scurvy was finally proven by American researcher Charles Glen King of the University of Pittsburgh. King's laboratory was given some hexuronic acid by Szent-Györgyi and soon established that it was the sought-after anti-scorbutic agent. Because of this, hexuronic acid was subsequently renamed *ascorbic acid.*

21st Century

In the 2010s, scurvy hasn't entirely disappeared from developed countries. Rates of incidence, while still very low, are increasing in the United Kingdom according to NHS Digital. Several cases were also reported in Westmead Hospital, Sydney, Australia.

Human Trials

Notable human dietary studies of experimentally induced scurvy have been conducted on conscientious objectors during WWII in Britain and on Iowa state prisoner volunteers in the late 1960s. These studies both found that all obvious symptoms of scurvy previously induced by an experimental scorbutic diet with extremely low vitamin C content could be completely reversed by additional vitamin C supplementation of only 10 mg per day. In these experiments, no clinical difference was noted between men given 70 mg vitamin C per day (which produced blood levels of vitamin C of about 0.55 mg/dl, about 1/3 of tissue saturation levels), and those given 10 mg per day (which produced lower blood levels). Men in the prison study developed the first signs of scurvy about 4 weeks after starting the vitamin C-free diet, whereas in the British study, six to eight months were required, possibly because the subjects were pre-loaded with a 70 mg/day supplement for six weeks before the scorbutic diet was fed.

Men in both studies, on a diet devoid or nearly devoid of vitamin C, had blood levels of vitamin C too low to be accurately measured when they developed signs of scurvy, and in the Iowa study, at this time were estimated (by labeled vitamin C dilution) to have a body pool of less than 300 mg, with daily turnover of only 2.5 mg/day.

Other Animals

Scurvy does not occur in most animals as they can make their own vitamin C. However, humans and other higher primates (the simians—monkeys and apes—and tarsiers), guinea pigs, most or all bats, and some species of birds and fish lack an enzyme (L-gulonolactone oxidase) necessary for such synthesis and must obtain vitamin C through their diet. The gene for L-gulonolactone oxidase is still present in the human genome, but deactivated by DNA mutations.

Almost all plant and animal species synthesize vitamin C. Notable mammalian exceptions include most or all of the order Chiroptera (bats), and one of the two major primate suborders, the “Anthropoidea” (Haplorrhini) which include tarsiers, monkeys, and apes, including human beings. The Strepsirrhini (non-tarsier prosimians) can make their own vitamin C, and these include lemurs, lorises, pottos, and galagos. Ascorbic acid is also not synthesized by at least two species of Caviidae, the capybara and the guinea pig. There are known species of birds and fish that do not synthesize their own Vitamin C. All species that do not synthesize ascorbate require it in the diet. Deficiency causes scurvy in humans, and somewhat similar symptoms in other animals.

Name

In babies, scurvy is sometimes referred to as Barlow’s disease, named after Thomas Barlow, a British physician who described it in 1883. However, Barlow’s disease may also refer to mitral valve prolapse.

Rickets

Rickets is defective mineralization or calcification of bones before epiphyseal closure in immature mammals due to deficiency or impaired metabolism of vitamin D, phosphorus or calcium, potentially leading to fractures and deformity. Rickets is among the most frequent childhood diseases in many developing countries. The predominant cause is a vitamin D deficiency, but lack of adequate calcium in the diet may also lead to rickets (cases of severe diarrhea and vomiting may be the cause of the deficiency). Although it can occur in adults, the majority of cases occur in children suffering from severe malnutrition, usually resulting from famine or starvation during the early stages of childhood.

Osteomalacia is a similar condition occurring in adults, generally due to a deficiency of vitamin D after epiphyseal closure.

Signs and Symptoms

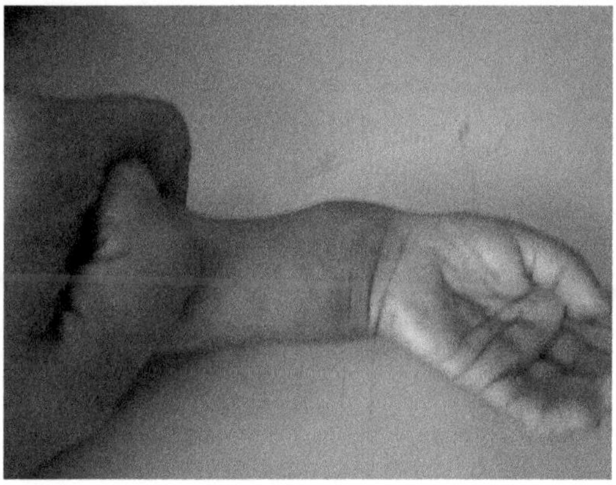

Widening of wrist

Signs and symptoms of rickets include:

- Bone tenderness
- Dental problems
- Muscle weakness (rickety myopathy)
- Increased tendency for fractures (easily broken bones), especially greenstick fractures
- Skeletal deformity
    - Toddlers: Bowed legs and double malleoli (genu varum)
    - Older children: Knock-knees (genu valgum) or “windswept knees”
    - Cranial deformity (such as skull bossing or delayed fontanelle closure)
    - Pelvic deformity
    - Pectus carinatum (“pigeon chest”)
    - Spinal deformity (such as kyphoscoliosis or lumbar lordosis)
- Growth disturbance
- Hypocalcemia (low level of calcium in the blood)
- Tetany (uncontrolled muscle spasms all over the body)
- Craniotabes (soft skull)
- Costochondral swelling (aka “rickety rosary” or “rachitic rosary”)

- Harrison's groove
- Double malleoli sign due to metaphyseal hyperplasia
- Widening of wrist raises early suspicion, it is due to metaphyseal cartilage hyperplasia.

An X-ray or radiograph of an advanced sufferer from rickets tends to present in a classic way: bow legs (outward curve of long bone of the legs) and a deformed chest. Changes in the skull also occur causing a distinctive "square headed" appearance (Caput Quadratum). These deformities persist into adult life if not treated. Long-term consequences include permanent bends or disfiguration of the long bones, and a curved back.

Cause

Maternal deficiencies may be the cause of overt bone disease from before birth and impairment of bone quality after birth. The primary cause of congenital rickets is vitamin D deficiency in the mother's blood, which the baby shares. Vitamin D ensures that serum phosphate and calcium levels are sufficient to facilitate the mineralization of bone. Congenital rickets may also be caused by other maternal diseases, including severe osteomalacia, untreated celiac disease, malabsorption, pre-eclampsia, and premature birth. Rickets in children is similar to osteoporosis in the elderly, with brittle bones. Pre-natal care includes checking vitamin levels and ensuring that any deficiencies are supplemented.

Also exclusively breast-fed infants may require rickets prevention by vitamin D supplementation or an increased exposure to sunlight.

In sunny countries such as Nigeria, South Africa, and Bangladesh, there is sufficient endogenous vitamin D due to exposure to the sun. However, the disease occurs among older toddlers and children in these countries, which in these circumstances is attributed to low dietary calcium intakes due to a mainly cereal-based diet.

Sunlight

Sunlight, especially ultraviolet light, lets human skin cells convert vitamin D from an inactive to active state. In the absence of vitamin D, dietary calcium is not properly absorbed, resulting in hypocalcaemia, leading to skeletal and dental deformities and neuromuscular symptoms, e.g. hyperexcitability. Foods that contain vitamin D include butter, eggs, fish liver oils, margarine, fortified milk and juice, portabella and shiitake mushrooms, and oily fishes such as tuna, herring, and salmon. A rare X-linked dominant form exists called vitamin D-resistant rickets or X-linked hypophosphatemia.

Cases have been reported in Britain in recent years of rickets in children of many social backgrounds caused by insufficient production in the body of vitamin D because the sun's ultraviolet light was not reaching the skin due to use of strong sunblock, too much "covering up" in sunlight, or not getting out into the sun. Other cases have been reported among the children of some ethnic groups in which mothers avoid exposure to the sun for religious or cultural reasons, leading to a maternal shortage of vitamin D; and people with darker skins need more sunlight to maintain vitamin D levels.

Rickets had historically been a problem in London, especially during the Industrial Revolution. Persistent thick fog and heavy industrial smog permeating the city blocked out significant amounts of sunlight to such an extent that up to 80 percent of children at one time had varying degrees of rickets in one form or the other.

Diseases causing soft bones in infants, like hypophosphatasia or hypophosphatemia can also lead to rickets.

Evolutionary Considerations

Vitamin D natural selection hypotheses: Rickets is often a result of Vitamin D3 deficiency. The Vitamin D natural selection hypothesis suggests that Vitamin D production from sunlight is a selective force for human skin color variation. The correlation between human skin color and latitude is thought to be the result of positive selection to varying levels of solar ultraviolet radiation. Northern latitudes have selection for lighter skin that allows UV rays to produce Vitamin D from 7-dehydrocholesterol. Conversely, latitudes near the equator have selection for darker skin that can block the majority of UV radiation to protect from toxic levels of Vitamin D, as well as skin cancer.

An anecdote often cited to support this hypothesis is that Arctic populations whose skin is relatively darker for their latitude, such as the Inuit, have a diet that is historically rich in vitamin D. Since these people acquire Vitamin D through their diet, there is not a positive selective force to synthesize Vitamin D from sunlight.

Environment mismatch: Ultimately, Vitamin D deficiency arises from a mismatch between a populations previous evolutionary environment and the individual's current environment. This risk of mismatch increases with advances in transportation methods and increases in urban population size at high latitudes.

Similar to the environmental mismatch when dark-skinned people live at high latitudes, Rickets can also occur in religious communities that require long garments with hoods and veils. These hoods and veils act as sunlight barriers that prevent individuals from synthesizing Vitamin D naturally from the sun.

In a study by Mithal et al., Vitamin D insufficiency of various countries was measured by lower 25-hydroxyvitamin D. 25(OH)D is an indicator of vitamin D insufficiency that can be easily measured. These percentages should be regarded as relative Vitamin D levels, and not as predicting evidence for development of rickets.

Asian immigrants living in Europe have an increased risk for Vitamin D deficiency. Vitamin D insufficiency was found in 40% of non-Western immigrants in the Netherlands, and in more than 80% of Turkish and Moroccan immigrants.

The Middle East, despite high rates of sun-exposure, has the highest rates of rickets worldwide. This can be explained by limited sun exposure due to cultural practices and lack of vitamin D supplementation for breast-feeding women. Up to 70% and 80% of adolescent girls in Iran and Saudi Arabia, respectively, have Vitamin D insufficiency. Socioeconomic factors that limit a Vitamin D rich diet also plays a role. In the United States, Vitamin D insufficiency varies dramatically by ethnicity. Among males aged 70 years and older, the prevalence of low serum 25(OH) D levels was 23% for non-Hispanic whites, 45% for Mexican Americans, and 58% for non-Hispanic blacks. Among women, the prevalence was 28.5%, 55%, and 68%, respectively.

A systematic review published in the Cochrane Library looked at children up to three years old in Turkey and China and found there was a negative association between vitamin D and rickets. In Turkey the kids getting vitamin D had only a 4% chance of developing rickets compared to the kids who received no medical intervention. In China, a combination of vitamin D, calcium and nutritional counseling was linked to a decreased risk of rickets.

With this evolutionary perspective in mind, parents can supplement their nutritional intake with vitamin D enhanced beverages if they feel their child is at risk for Vitamin D deficiency, or, with more assurance of benefit and no cost, enable the child to spend more time with some of their skin receiving the summer sun's rays.

Diagnosis

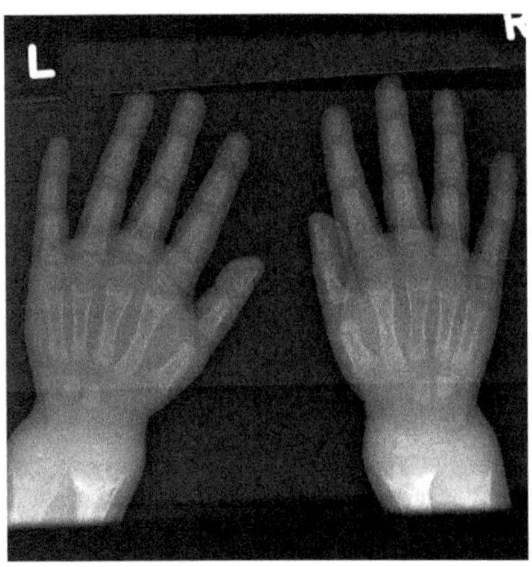

Wrist X ray showing changes in rickets. Mainly cupping is seen here.

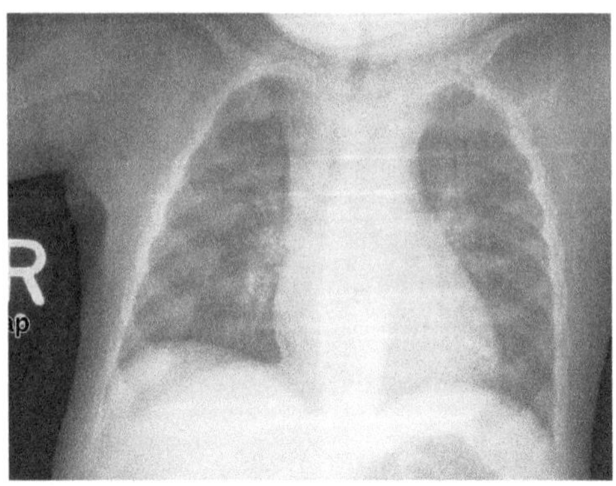

Chest X ray showing changes consistent with rickets. These changes are usually referred to as "rosary beads" of rickets.

Rickets may be diagnosed with the help of:

- Blood tests:
    - Serum calcium may show low levels of calcium, serum phosphorus may be low, and serum alkaline phosphatase may be high from bones or changes in the shape or structure of the bones. This can show enlarged limbs and joints.
- Bone biopsy is rarely performed but will confirm rickets.

Types

- Vitamin D-related rickets
    - Vitamin D deficiency
    - Vitamin D-dependent rickets
        - Type 1 (25-Hydroxyvitamin D3 1-alpha-hydroxylase deficiency)
        - Type 2 (calcitriol receptor mutation)
- Hypocalcemia-related rickets
    - Hypocalcemia
    - Chronic renal failure (CKD-BMD)
- Hypophosphatemia-related rickets
    - Congenital
        - Vitamin D-resistant rickets
        - Autosomal dominant hypophosphatemic rickets (ADHR)
        - Autosomal recessive hypophosphatemic rickets (ARHR)
    - Hypophosphatemia (typically secondary to malabsorption)
    - Fanconi's syndrome
- Secondary to other diseases
    - Tumor-induced osteomalacia
    - McCune-Albright syndrome
    - Epidermal nevus syndrome
    - Dent's disease

Differential Diagnosis

Infants with rickets often have bone fractures. This sometimes leads to child abuse allegations. This issue appears to be more common for solely nursing infants of black mothers, in winter in temperate climates, suffering poor nutrition and no vitamin D supplementation. People with darker skin produce less vitamin D than those with lighter skin, for the same amount of sunlight.

Treatment and Prevention

The most common treatment of rickets is the use of Vitamin D. However, surgery may be required to remove severe bone abnormalities.

Diet and Sunlight

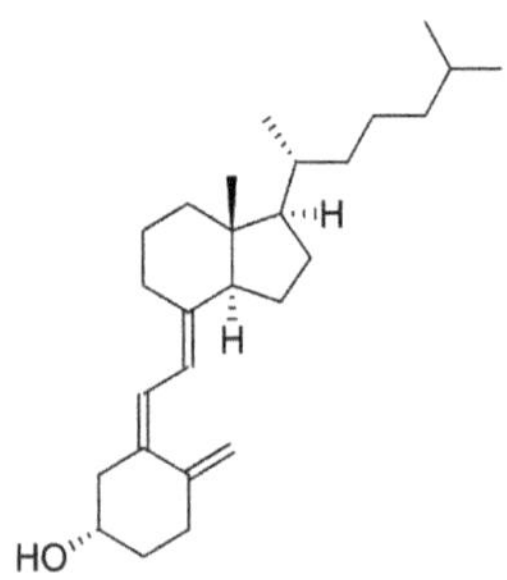

Cholecalciferol (D_3)

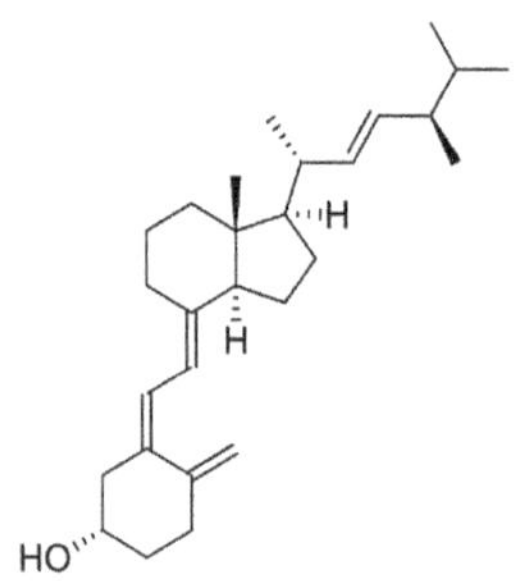

Ergocalciferol (D_2)

Treatment involves increasing dietary intake of calcium, phosphates and vitamin D. Exposure to ultraviolet B light (most easily obtained when the sun is highest in the sky), cod liver oil, halibut-liver oil, and viosterol are all sources of vitamin D.

A sufficient amount of ultraviolet B light in sunlight each day and adequate supplies of calcium and phosphorus in the diet can prevent rickets. Darker-skinned people need to be exposed longer to the ultraviolet rays. The replacement of vitamin D has been proven to correct rickets using these methods of ultraviolet light therapy and medicine.

Recommendations are for 400 international units (IU) of vitamin D a day for infants and children. Children who do not get adequate amounts of vitamin D are at increased risk of rickets. Vitamin D is essential for allowing the body to uptake calcium for use in proper bone calcification and maintenance.

Supplementation

Sufficient vitamin D levels can also be achieved through dietary supplementation and/or exposure to sunlight. Vitamin D_3 (cholecalciferol) is the preferred form since it is more readily absorbed than vitamin D_2. Most dermatologists recommend vitamin D supplementation as an alternative to unprotected ultraviolet exposure due to the increased risk of skin cancer associated with sun exposure. Endogenous production with full body exposure to sunlight is approximately 250 µg (10,000 IU) per day.

According to the American Academy of Pediatrics (AAP), all infants, including those who are exclusively breast-fed, may need Vitamin D supplementation until they start drinking at least 17 US fluid ounces (500 ml) of vitamin D-fortified milk or formula a day.

Epidemiology

In developed countries, rickets is a rare disease (incidence of less than 1 in 200,000). Recently, cases of rickets have been reported among children who are fed plant-based milk substitutes and not given supplemental vitamin D.

Those at higher risk for developing rickets include:

- Breast-fed infants whose mothers are not exposed to sunlight
- Breast-fed infants who are not exposed to sunlight
- Breast-fed babies who are exposed to little sunlight
- Adolescents, in particular when undergoing the pubertal growth spurt
- Any child whose diet does not contain enough vitamin D or calcium

History

Greek physician Soranus of Ephesus, one of the chief representatives of the Methodic school of medicine who practiced in Alexandria and subsequently in Rome, reported deformation of the bones in infants as early as the first and second centuries AD. Rickets was not defined as a specific medical condition until 1645, when an English physician Daniel Whistler gave the earliest known description of the disease. In 1650 a treatise on rickets was published by Francis Glisson, a physician at Caius College, Cambridge, who said it had first appeared about 30 years previously in the counties of Dorset and Somerset. In 1857, John Snow suggested rickets, then widespread in Britain, was being caused by the adulteration of bakers' bread with alum. German pediatrician Kurt Huldschinsky successfully demonstrated in the winter of 1918–1919 how rickets could be treated with ultraviolet lamps. The role of diet in the development of rickets was determined by Edward Mellanby between 1918–1920. In 1923, American physician Harry Steenbock demonstrated that irradiation by ultraviolet light increased the vitamin D content of foods and other organic materials. Steenbock's irradiation technique was used for food stuffs, but most memorably for milk. By 1945, rickets had all but been eliminated in the United States, no cases have been recorded in Cuba, but they are there since the Special Period.

Etymology

The word *rickets* may be from the Old English word *wrickken* ('to twist'), although because this is conjectured, several major dictionaries simply say "origin unknown". The name *rickets* is plural in form but usually singular in construction. The Greek word "rachitis" (meaning "in or of the spine") was later adopted as the scientific term for rickets, due chiefly to the words' similarity in sound.

In Dutch and German rickets is known as "English disease"

References

- Ellis CN, Vanderveen EE, Rasmussen JE (1984). "Scurvy. A case caused by peculiar dietary habits". Arch Dermatol. 120 (9): 1212–4. PMID 6476860. doi:10.1001/archderm.120.9.1212
- Itokawa, Yoshinori (1976). "Kanehiro Takaki (1849–1920): A Biographical Sketch". Journal of Nutrition. 106 (5): 581–8. PMID 772183
- Vetreno, Ryan Peter (2011). Thiamine deficiency-induced neurodegeneration and neurogenesis (PhD Thesis). Binghampton University. ISBN 978-1-124-75696-7. OCLC 781626781
- Feibel, Carrie (2016-08-15). "The Return of Scurvy? Houston Neurologist Diagnoses Hundreds of Patients with Vitamin Deficiencies". Houston Public Media. University of Houston. Retrieved 2016-08-17.
- Kopelman, M. D.; Thomson, A. D.; Guerrini, I.; Marshall, E. J. (2009). "The Korsakoff Syndrome: Clinical Aspects, Psychology and Treatment". Alcohol and Alcoholism. 44 (2): 148–54. PMID 19151162. doi:10.1093/alcalc/agn118
- Davies IJ, Temperley JM (1967). "A case of scurvy in a student". Postgraduate Medical Journal. 43 (502): 549–50. PMC 2466190 . PMID 6074157. doi:10.1136/pgmj.43.502.539
- Merle A. Carter & Edward Bernstein (2005). "Acute and Chronic Alcohol Intoxication". In Elizabeth Mitchell & Ron Medzon. Introduction to Emergency Medicine. Lippincott Williams & Wilkins. p. 272. ISBN 978-0-7817-3200-0
- Croucher, Martin (September 19, 2012). "Dubai boy, 4, suffers scurvy after meat-only diet". The National (Abu Dhabi). Retrieved 5 October 2012
- Harper, Clive; Fornes, Paul; Duyckaerts, Charles; Lecomte, Dominique; Hauw, Jean-Jacques (1995). "An international perspective on the prevalence of the Wernicke-Korsakoff syndrome". Metabolic Brain Disease. 10 (1): 17–24. PMID 7596325. doi:10.1007/BF01991779
- Bartholomew, Michael (2002). "James Lind and scurvy: A revaluation". Journal for Maritime Research. 4 (1): 1–14. PMID 20355298. doi:10.1080/21533369.2002.9668317. Retrieved February 16, 2015
- Berg, Jeremy M; Tymoczko, John L; Stryer, Lubert (2002). "The Disruption of Pyruvate Metabolism Is the Cause of Beriberi and Poisoning by Mercury and Arsenic". Biochemistry (5th ed.). ISBN 978-0-7167-3051-4
- Hodges, R. E.; Baker, E. M.; Hood, J.; Sauberlich, H. E.; March, S. C. (1969). "Experimental Scurvy in Man". American Journal of Clinical Nutrition. 22 (5): 535–548. PMID 4977512
- Lamb, Jonathan (2001). Preserving the self in the south seas, 1680–1840. University of Chicago Press. p. 117. ISBN 0-226-46849-6

- Higdon, Jane, Ph.D. (2006-01-31). "Vitamin C". Oregon State University, Micronutrient Information Center. Retrieved 2007-03-07
- Donnino M (2004). "Gastrointestinal Beriberi: A Previously Unrecognized Syndrome". Ann Intern Med. 141: 898–899. doi:10.7326/0003-4819-141-11-200412070-00035
- Balasubramanian S, Ganesh R (2008). "Vitamin D deficiency in exclusively breast-fed infants". The Indian Journal of Medical Research (Review). 127 (3): 250–5. PMID 18497439
- McKenna KE, Dawson JF (1993). "Scurvy occurring in a teenager". Clin. Exp. Dermatol. 18 (1): 75–7. PMID 8440062. doi:10.1111/j.1365-2230.1993.tb00976.x
- Fernandez-Armesto, Felipe (2006). Pathfinders: A Global History of Exploration. W.W. Norton & Company. pp. 297–298. ISBN 0-393-06259-7
- THE MIDDLE EAST & AFRICA REGIONAL AUDIT, Executive Summary, Epidemiology, costs & burden of osteoporosis in 2011, The International Osteoporosis Foundation, www.iofbonehealth.org, retrieved 6 April 2017
- Sechi, G; Serra, A (May 2007). "Wernicke's encephalopathy: new clinical settings and recent advances in diagnosis and management". Lancet neurology. 6 (5): 442–55. PMID 17434099. doi:10.1016/S1474-4422(07)70104-7

Permissions

All chapters in this book are published with permission under the Creative Commons Attribution Share Alike License or equivalent. Every chapter published in this book has been scrutinized by our experts. Their significance has been extensively debated. The topics covered herein carry significant information for a comprehensive understanding. They may even be implemented as practical applications or may be referred to as a beginning point for further studies.

We would like to thank the editorial team for lending their expertise to make the book truly unique. They have played a crucial role in the development of this book. Without their invaluable contributions this book wouldn't have been possible. They have made vital efforts to compile up to date information on the varied aspects of this subject to make this book a valuable addition to the collection of many professionals and students.

This book was conceptualized with the vision of imparting up-to-date and integrated information in this field. To ensure the same, a matchless editorial board was set up. Every individual on the board went through rigorous rounds of assessment to prove their worth. After which they invested a large part of their time researching and compiling the most relevant data for our readers.

The editorial board has been involved in producing this book since its inception. They have spent rigorous hours researching and exploring the diverse topics which have resulted in the successful publishing of this book. They have passed on their knowledge of decades through this book. To expedite this challenging task, the publisher supported the team at every step. A small team of assistant editors was also appointed to further simplify the editing procedure and attain best results for the readers.

Apart from the editorial board, the designing team has also invested a significant amount of their time in understanding the subject and creating the most relevant covers. They scrutinized every image to scout for the most suitable representation of the subject and create an appropriate cover for the book.

The publishing team has been an ardent support to the editorial, designing and production team. Their endless efforts to recruit the best for this project, has resulted in the accomplishment of this book. They are a veteran in the field of academics and their pool of knowledge is as vast as their experience in printing. Their expertise and guidance has proved useful at every step. Their uncompromising quality standards have made this book an exceptional effort. Their encouragement from time to time has been an inspiration for everyone.

The publisher and the editorial board hope that this book will prove to be a valuable piece of knowledge for students, practitioners and scholars across the globe.

Index